I0465564

PUBLISHER COMMENTARY

This PRINT REPLICA contains the FDA guidance for industry on **Distributing Scientific and Medical Publications on Unapproved New Uses** dated February 2014, and the **Food and Drug Administration Modernization Act of 1997**.

This is a revision of the guidance released in 2009 and is intended to clarify the ways in which a medical device manufacturer or pharmaceutical company or may use scientific and medical literature to promote its products, even if the literature doesn't conform to the FDA-approved uses for the product. This is a checklist that companies will need to consult for each instance of scientific and medical literature they wish to promote. These include medical and promotional interactions with health care professionals (HCP), Payer/Formulary Access Interactions, Publications, Grants And Continuing Medical Education (CME), Investigator Initiated Studies (IIS), and Post-Marketing Studies.

According to the Executive Director of the Coalition for Healthcare Communication, John Kamp, "Manufacturers should be able to distribute truthful information – in the form of journal articles, medical textbooks and practice guidelines." (Publisher comment: It's called FREE SPEECH).

Why buy a hard copy book you can download for free?

We print this so you don't have to.

Anyone that has worked in this industry knows how difficult it is to search for that one bit of information that will make or break a deal. Many people need glasses to read and don't like books with small print. That's especially true of complex technical subjects like acquisition regulations. We print the hard copy books a full 8 ½ inches by 11 inches, with large text. There are also wide margins so you can jot down notes.

You could print a 1,900-page book over the network, punch holes and put it in a humongous binder, but it's not cost effective. A contracting officer that's paid $75 an hour has to do this using a printer shared with 100 other people – and it's out of paper, and the toner is low. It's much easier to order a copy at Amazon.com

This material is published by 4th Watch Publishing Co. We publish tightly-bound, full-size books at 8 ½ by 11 inches, with large text and glossy covers. 4th Watch Publishing Co. is a Service Disabled Veteran Owned Small Business (SDVOSB). Please visit www.usgovpub.com.

Other books we publish that are available on Amazon.com include:

GAO	Principles of Federal Appropriations Law
GAO FAM	GAO Financial Audit Manual
GAO-01-1008G	Internal Control Management and Evaluation Tool
GAO-17-313SP	Government Auditing Standards (Yellow Book)
GAO-14-704G	Standards for Internal Control in the Federal Government (Green Book)
FISCAM	Federal Information System Controls Audit Manual
OMB A-123	Management's Responsibility for Enterprise Risk Management and Internal Control
FISMA	Federal Information Security Modernization Act & OMB A-130
FY19 Budget	Budget of the U.S. Government
FITARA	Federal Information Technology Acquisition Reform

Federal Rules of Appellate Procedure (2017)
Federal Rules of Rules of Criminal Procedure (2017)
Federal Rules of Rules of Civil Procedure (2017)
Federal Rules of Rules of Bankruptcy Procedure (2017)
Benchbook for U.S. District Court Judges (2013)
Military Judges' Benchbook (2017)
Principles of Federal Appropriations Law 4th Edition
Immigration Court Practice Manual
DoD Law of War Manual (2016)
DoD Operational Law Handbook (2017)
DoD Domestic Operational Law Handbook (2015)
DoD Rule of Law Handbook (2015)

Distributing Scientific and Medical Publications on Unapproved New Uses — Recommended Practices

REVISED DRAFT GUIDANCE

This guidance document is being distributed for comment purposes only.

Comments and suggestions regarding this draft document should be submitted within 60 days of publication in the *Federal Register* of the notice announcing the availability of the draft guidance. Submit electronic comments to http://www.regulations.gov. Submit written comments to the Division of Dockets Management (HFA-305), Food and Drug Administration, 5630 Fishers Lane, rm. 1061, Rockville, MD 20852. All comments should be identified with the docket number listed in the notice of availability that publishes in the *Federal Register*.

For questions regarding this draft document contact (CDER) Bryant Godfrey at 301-796-1200, (CBER) the Office of Communication, Outreach and Development at 301-827-1800, or (CDRH) Deborah Wolf at 301-796-5732.

U.S. Department of Health and Human Services
Food and Drug Administration
Center for Drug Evaluation and Research (CDER)
Center for Biologics Evaluation and Research (CBER)
Center for Devices and Radiological Health (CDRH)

February 2014
Procedural

Distributing Scientific and Medical Publications on Unapproved New Uses—Recommended Practices

Additional copies are available from:

Office of Communications
Division of Drug Information, WO51, Room 2201
Center for Drug Evaluation and Research
Food and Drug Administration
10903 New Hampshire Ave., Silver Spring, MD 20993
Phone: 301-796-3400; Fax: 301-847-8714
http://www.fda.gov/Drugs/GuidanceComplianceRegulatoryInformation/Guidances/default.htm
Email: druginfo@fda.hhs.gov
and/or
Office of Communication, Outreach and
Development, HFM-40
Center for Biologics Evaluation and Research
Food and Drug Administration
1401 Rockville Pike, Rockville, MD 20852-1448
Phone: 800-835-4709 or 301-827-1800
http://www.fda.gov/BiologicsBloodVaccines/GuidanceComplianceRegulatoryInformation/Guidances/default.htm
Email: ocod@fda.hhs.gov
and/or
Office of Communication, Education and Radiation Programs
Division of Small Manufacturers Assistance, WO66-4613
Center for Devices and Radiological Health
Food and Drug Administration
10903 New Hampshire Ave., Silver Spring, MD 20993
Fax: 301.847.8149
Manufacturers Assistance Phone: 800.638.2041 or 301.796.7100
International Staff Phone: 301.827.3993
http://www.fda.gov/MedicalDevices/DeviceRegulationandGuidance/GuidanceDocuments/default.htm
Email: dsmica@cdrh.fda.gov

U.S. Department of Health and Human Services
Food and Drug Administration
Center for Drug Evaluation and Research (CDER)
Center for Biologics Evaluation and Research (CBER)
Center for Devices and Radiological Health (CDRH)

February 2014
Procedural

TABLE OF CONTENTS

1
2

Distributing Scientific and Medical Publications on Unapproved New Uses — Recommended Practices[1]

3
4
5

> This draft guidance, when finalized, will represent the Food and Drug Administration's (FDA's) current thinking on this topic. It does not create or confer any rights for or on any person and does not operate to bind FDA or the public. You can use an alternative approach if the approach satisfies the requirements of the applicable statutes and regulations. If you want to discuss an alternative approach, contact the FDA staff responsible for implementing this guidance. If you cannot identify the appropriate FDA staff, call the appropriate number listed on the title page of this guidance.

6
7
8
9
10
11
12
13
14
15

16 I.   INTRODUCTION

17
18 This guidance describes the Food and Drug Administration's (FDA's or Agency's) current
19 thinking on recommended practices for drug and medical device manufacturers and their
20 representatives[2] to follow when distributing to health care professionals or health care entities[3]
21 scientific or medical journal articles, scientific or medical reference texts, or clinical practice
22 guidelines (CPGs) that discuss unapproved new uses[4] for approved drugs or approved or cleared
23 medical devices[5] marketed in the United States. For the purposes of this guidance, these
24 materials are generally referred to as *scientific and medical publications*.
25

---

[1] This guidance was developed by the Center for Drug Evaluation and Research (CDER) in collaboration with the Center for Biologics Evaluation and Research (CBER) and the Center for Devices and Radiological Health (CDRH) in the Food and Drug Administration.

[2] As used in this guidance, *manufacturer* means a person who manufactures a drug or device or who is licensed by such person to distribute or market the drug or device, or a representative of such a person. The term might also include the sponsor of the approved, licensed, cleared, or 510(k) exempt drug or device.

[3] As used in this guidance, *health care entity* includes hospitals, professional medical organizations, drug formulary committees, pharmacy benefits managers, health insurance issuers, group health plans, and Federal or State governmental agencies involved in the provision of health care or health insurance.

[4] The terms *unapproved new use*, *unapproved use*, and *off-label use* are used interchangeably in this guidance to refer to a use of an approved or cleared medical product that is not included in the product's approved labeling or cleared indications for use statement. Although this guidance focuses on unapproved uses of approved and cleared medical products, the recommendations in this guidance also apply to manufacturer distribution of publications that discuss unapproved new uses that are not included in the exemption from premarket notification for those class I or class II devices that are otherwise exempt from the requirement to submit a 510(k).

[5] As used in this guidance, the terms *drug* and *device* refer to drugs and devices intended for use in humans, and include biological products licensed under section 351(a) of the Public Health Service (PHS) Act (42 U.S.C. 262(a)). *See* 42 U.S.C. 262(j). Different provisions govern the use of drugs in animals, which are not generally addressed in this guidance. *See* sections 512(a)(4) and (a)(5) of the Food, Drug & Cosmetic Act and this Agency's regulations at 21 CFR part 530 for specific provisions related to the off-label (or extra-label) use of approved animal and human drugs in animals.

26   In 2009, FDA issued a guidance titled *Good Reprint Practices for the Distribution of Medical*
27   *Journal Articles and Medical or Scientific Reference Publications on Unapproved New Uses of*
28   *Approved Drugs and Approved or Cleared Medical Devices* (2009 guidance) to provide
29   guidance on manufacturer distribution of "journal articles" and "scientific or medical reference
30   publications." FDA is revising its 2009 guidance on good reprint practices to clarify the
31   Agency's position on manufacturer dissemination of scientific or medical reference texts and
32   CPGs that include information on unapproved new uses of the manufacturer's products. New
33   explanatory sections have been included on these topics. This revised draft guidance is being
34   issued to enable the public to provide comments.
35
36   FDA's guidance documents, including this draft guidance, do not establish legally enforceable
37   rights or responsibilities. Instead, guidances describe the Agency's current thinking on a topic
38   and should be viewed only as recommendations, unless specific regulatory or statutory
39   requirements are cited. The use of the word *should* in Agency guidances means that something
40   is suggested or recommended, but not required.
41
42   Similarly, the use of *should not* in this guidance does not suggest or create an independent legal
43   prohibition, but indicates recommended practice.
44
45   **II.   BACKGROUND**
46
47   The evolution of drug and medical device regulation in the United States has been shaped by
48   experience with the real and substantial risks to the public from uses of drugs and medical
49   devices not shown to be both safe and effective through adequate and well-controlled clinical
50   studies. While physicians may exercise their professional judgment to make individual patient
51   care decisions, the public health often is not well served when those judgments rest on anecdotal
52   experience or even preliminary scientific study—too often, the promise of safety and
53   effectiveness made by such sources has not been demonstrated when adequate and well-
54   controlled clinical studies are completed.[6]
55
56   These public health concerns are not limited to drugs and medical devices that lack FDA
57   approval or clearance for any use. These concerns are also relevant to new intended uses for
58   previously approved or cleared medical products, given that approval of a drug or medical device

---

[6] *See, e.g.*, Echt DS, Liebson PR, Mitchell LB et al., "Mortality and Morbidity in Patients Receiving Encainide, Flecainide, or Placebo: The Cardiac Arrhythmia Suppression Trial," *New Eng. J. Med.*, 324(12): 781-88 (1991). The Cardiac Arrhythmia Suppression Trial (CAST) examined the widely held belief (in the absence of well-controlled studies showing this to be true) that treating minor rhythm abnormalities (frequent ventricular premature beats) with anti-arrhythmics after an acute myocardial infarction would improve survival. The well-controlled study (CAST) to test this belief, conducted by the National Institutes of Health, demonstrated that, although the drugs did indeed treat minor rhythm abnormalities, the patients who took those drugs had a 2 ½ fold increase in mortality. *See also* National Academy of Sciences, "Drug Efficacy Study: Final Report to the Commissioner of Food and Drugs, Food and Drug Administration" (1969), which found that approximately one-third of all pre-1962 marketed drugs did not have a single effective use.

59 for one intended use does not assure its safety and effectiveness for other uses.[7] A separate
60 balancing of risks and benefits is necessary for each intended use.[8]
61
62 For these reasons, the modern Federal Food, Drug, and Cosmetic Act (FD&C Act) and FDA
63 regulations prohibit manufacturers from introducing new drugs and most class III medical
64 devices into interstate commerce for any intended use that FDA has not determined to be safe
65 and effective.[9] These authorities also prohibit manufacturers from introducing into interstate
66 commerce devices subject to premarket notification requirements under section 510(k), which
67 includes most class II and some class I devices, for any intended use that is outside FDA's
68 substantial equivalence determination (clearance) for such devices.[10] Devices that are exempt
69 from premarket notification requirements, generally because they are low risk, may be
70 introduced into interstate commerce for the specifically exempt intended use(s) without
71 obtaining FDA clearance.[11] To establish a manufacturer's or distributor's intended use for the
72 product, FDA is not bound by the manufacturer's or distributor's subjective claims of intent, but

---

[7] Indeed, Congress added the concept of effectiveness to the Food, Drug, and Cosmetic Act's (FD&C Act's) definition of "new drug" (and not merely to other provisions of the FD&C Act) to prevent manufacturers from obtaining approval of a drug for one use, and then marketing the drug for unapproved, or "off-label," uses. *See* S. Rep. No. 87-1744 (1962), reprinted in 1962 U.S.C.C.A.N. 2884, 2901-2903 (statement of Senators Kefauver, Carroll, Dodd, Hart & Long, explaining reasons for changing the definition of "new drug"). As Senator Kefauver explained, if a manufacturer were not required to demonstrate safety and effectiveness for each new intended use, "[t]he expectation would be that the initial claims would tend to be quite limited." *Id*. Then, once the drug was approved for one use, "'the sky would be the limit' and extreme claims of any kind could be made . . . ." *Id*. Similar requirements were subsequently extended to medical devices.

[8] *See, e.g.*, United States v. Rutherford, 442 U.S. 544, 555 (1979) ("Few if any drugs are completely safe in the sense that they may be taken by all persons in all circumstances without risk. Thus, the Commissioner generally considers a drug safe when the expected therapeutic gain justifies the risk entailed by its use"); Rhone-Poulenc, Inc. v. FDA, 636 F. 2d 750, 752 (D.C. Cir. 1980).

[9] *See, e.g.*, sections, 505(a), 515 (a), 501(f)(1), and 301(a) and (d), of the FD&C Act (21 U.S.C. 355(a), 360e(a), 351(f)(1)) and 331(a) and (d). The requirement that safety and effectiveness for each intended use be established before introduction of the product into interstate commerce for that use came from experience showing that exclusive reliance on post-hoc remedies, such as enforcement actions for false or misleading labeling, was inadequate to protect the public health, as these remedies were not sufficient to deter manufacturers and distributors—who profit from sales of their products for any use—from making unsubstantiated and misleading claims to encourage use of their products. As the Secretary of Health, Education, and Welfare told Congress, "[i]t is intolerable to permit the marketing of worthless products under the rules of a cat-and-mouse-game where a manufacturer can fool the public until the [FDA] finally catches up with him." *The Drug Industry Antitrust Act of 1962: Hearings before the Antitrust Subcomm. of the Comm. on the Judiciary*, 87th Cong., 2d Sess. 173 (1962).

[10] *See* sections 502(o), 501(f)(1), 513(f)(1), 515, and 301(a) and (d) of the FD&C Act (21 U.S.C. 352(o), 351(f)(1), 360c(f)(1), 360e and 331(a) and (d)).

[11] *See* sections 510(l) and (m) of the FD&C Act (21 U.S.C. 360(l) and (m)).

73 rather can present objective evidence, which may include a variety of direct and circumstantial
74 evidence.[12]
75
76 Under the FD&C Act, an approved new drug that is accompanied by written, printed, or graphic
77 matter that suggests an unapproved use may be an unapproved new drug with respect to that
78 use.[13] Furthermore, an approved prescription drug that is intended for an unapproved use
79 (whether referenced in labeling or not) would be considered misbranded, because the drug does
80 not meet the regulatory exemptions from the requirement that its labeling bear "adequate
81 directions for use."[14] Similarly, a medical device that is intended for an unapproved use is
82 considered adulterated and misbranded.[15]
83

---

[12] *See, e.g.*, Action on Smoking and Health v. Harris, 655 F. 2d 236, 239 (D.C. Cir. 1980) (observing that "it is well established that the 'intended use' of a product, within the meaning of the [Food, Drug, and Cosmetic] Act is determined from its label, accompanying labeling, promotional claims, advertising and any other relevant source"); Hanson v. United States, 417 F. Supp. 30, 35 (D. Minn.), aff'd, 540 F. 2d 947 (8th Cir. 1976) (same); United States v. Travia, 180 F. Supp. 2d 115, 119 (D.D.C. 2001) (holding that "labeling is not exclusive evidence of the seller's intent," and finding nitrous oxide to be a drug from the circumstances of its sale, even where no labeling or oral statements accompanied product); United States v. Undetermined Quantities of Articles of Drug, 145 F. Supp. 2d 692, 698-99 (D. Md. 2001) (stating that "[o]f primary significance in determining whether a product may be deemed a 'drug' is its intended use or effect as gathered from the objective evidence disseminated by the vendor" and finding product to be drug where, among other things, marketing suggested that product was substitute for illegal drugs); United States v. 250 Jars, Etc. of U.S. Fancy Pure Honey, 218 F. Supp. 208, 211 (E.D. Mich. 1963) (finding distribution of pamphlets and newspaper articles containing claims for the curative power of honey by seller of honey to be evidence of intended use that rendered the seller's honey a drug); 21 C.F.R. §§ 201.128 (defining indicia of "intended use" for drugs); 801.4 (defining indicia of "intended use" for devices).

[13] *See* sections 201(m) and (p) of the FD&C Act, 21 U.S.C. 321 (m) and (p). Introducing an unapproved new drug into interstate commerce is prohibited. Sections 505(a) and 301(d) of the FD&C Act (21 U.S.C. 355(a) and 331(d)).

[14] *See* section 502(f) of the FD&C Act (21 U.S.C. 352(f)) and 21 CFR 201.5, 201.100(c)(1), and 201.115. Under section 502(f) and 21 C.F.R. 201.5, all drugs must bear directions under which a layperson can use the drug safely for each of its intended uses. Prescription drugs may be exempt from this requirement, and thus avoid being misbranded under section 502(f), if they satisfy the exemption from "adequate directions for use" in 21 CFR 201.100. That regulation, among other things, requires that the labeling of a prescription drug "bear adequate information for its use . . . under which practitioners licensed by law to administer the drug can use the drug safely and for the purposes for which it is intended, including all purposes for which it is advertised or represented." Further, if the prescription drug is subject to the new drug approval requirements of section 505 of the FD&C Act, the labeling containing this information must be the labeling authorized by an approved new drug application. The regulations further state that new drugs shall be exempt from section 502(f)(1) of the Act (21 U.S.C. 352(f)(1)) to the extent the exemption is claimed in an application approved under sections 505 or 512 of the Act. This exemption cannot be claimed, however, by a drug that would be a "new drug" if its labeling bore representations for its intended uses. *See* 21 CFR 201.115.

[15] *See* sections 501(f)(1), 502(o), 513(f)(1), and 515 of the FD&C Act (21 U.S.C. 351(f)(1), 352(o)), 360c(f)(1), and 360e).

84 As Congress recognized, starting with the Kefauver-Harris Amendments in 1962,[16] requiring
85 each new indication and intended use of a product to be approved or cleared by FDA is critical to
86 the protection of the public health. FDA regulatory processes not only ensure that each use of a
87 drug or medical device is supported by appropriate scientific evidence, but also that this
88 scientific information is used to develop labeling to support the safe and effective use of each
89 product.[17] Such labeling is in turn required to be provided with the product. Distribution of
90 scientific and medical publications regarding a medical product is not a substitute for the
91 information contained in FDA-approved product labeling.
92
93 In 1997, Congress passed the Food and Drug Administration Modernization Act (FDAMA).[18]
94 Section 401 of FDAMA[19] described certain conditions under which a drug or medical device
95 manufacturer could choose to disseminate medical and scientific information that discusses
96 unapproved uses of approved drugs and cleared or approved medical devices to "health care
97 professionals and certain entities, including pharmacy benefits managers, health insurance
98 issuers, group health plans, and Federal or State governmental agencies," without such
99 dissemination being considered as evidence of the manufacturer's intent that the product be used
100 for an unapproved new use. Among those conditions was the expectation that the manufacturer
101 of the product would seek FDA approval for the unapproved new use referenced in the
102 disseminated literature. With this condition, Congress again recognized the important public
103 health value of FDA premarket review and approval.
104
105 FDA's implementing regulations for section 401 of FDAMA were codified at 21 CFR part 99.
106 Section 401 of FDAMA included a sunset date of September 30, 2006. This statutory provision,
107 as well as FDA's pre-FDAMA guidance documents regarding reprint distribution and
108 manufacturer sponsorship of continuing medical education, was challenged on First Amendment
109 grounds. Although the district court found section 401 of FDAMA to be unconstitutional, the
110 U.S. Court of Appeals ultimately vacated the lower court's decision.[20]
111
112 In 2000, following the U.S. Court of Appeals ruling, FDA published a notice[21] confirming that
113 the provisions of section 401 of FDAMA and FDA's implementing regulations would continue
114 to apply. In that notice, FDA also stated that the statute and implementing regulations had

---

[16] *See* Pub.L. No. 87-781, 76 Stat. 780 (1962) ("Kefauver-Harris Amendments"); see footnote 7, above. Among other things, the Kefauver-Harris Amendments added the requirement that manufacturers demonstrate that their new drugs are effective, as well as safe, for their intended uses *before* they could be distributed. *See* 21 U.S.C. § 355(a), (d); *see also*, 21 U.S.C. 360e(a), (d) (requiring proof of safety and effectiveness for premarket approval of class III devices). As mentioned in footnote 7, the Kefauver-Harris Amendments also revised the FD&C Act's "new drug" definition to provide that a drug is a new drug if it is not generally recognized as "safe and effective" for its intended uses. *Id.* § 321(p). Because a drug is a "new drug" if it is not generally recognized as safe and effective for each intended use, a new intended use renders an approved drug a "new drug" with respect to the new use, and the manufacturer cannot distribute the drug in interstate commerce for that use without first obtaining FDA's approval of an application that demonstrates the drug's safety and effectiveness for the new use. *See* Washington Legal Foundation v. Henney, 202 F. 3d 331, 332-33 (D.C. Cir. 2000) ("it is unlawful for a manufacturer to introduce a drug into interstate commerce with an intent that it be used for an off-label purpose").
[17] *See* section 502(f)(1) of the Act; *see also, e.g.,* 21 CFR 201.100; 21 CFR 801.109.
[18] Pub. L. No. 105-115, 111 Stat. 2296.
[19] *See* section 551 of the FD&C Act (21 U.S.C. 360aaa).
[20] *See* Henney, 202 F. 3d 331.
[21] *See* 65 FR 14286, March 16, 2000.

115   constituted a "safe harbor" for a manufacturer that complied with them before and while
116   disseminating "journal articles and reference texts" about unapproved new uses of approved or
117   cleared products. The notice explained that if a manufacturer complied with the FDAMA
118   provisions, distributing such journal articles or reference texts would not have been used as
119   evidence of intent that the product distributed by the manufacturer be used for an unapproved
120   use. The notice clarified further that even if a manufacturer chose to disseminate materials in a
121   way that was inconsistent with section 401 of FDAMA, that dissemination would not be treated
122   as an independent violation of the law, but could have been used as evidence of a manufacturer's
123   intent that the product be used for an unapproved use.
124

125   On September 30, 2006, section 401 of FDAMA sunset and the implementing regulations in 21
126   CFR part 99 ceased to be applicable. In the wake of the sunset of the legislation, FDA issued
127   guidance, finalized in 2009, on good reprint practices. The 2009 guidance was intended to
128   provide drug and medical device manufacturers and their representatives with recommendations
129   on distributing scientific or medical information on unapproved uses to health care professionals
130   and health care entities, without such dissemination being considered as evidence of the
131   manufacturer's intent that the product be used for an unapproved new use.
132

133   The 2009 guidance, consistent with the objectives of section 401 of FDAMA (which was no
134   longer law), recognized that the public health may benefit when health care professionals receive
135   truthful and non-misleading scientific or medical publications on unapproved new uses.[22] This
136   information can be particularly important given that a health care professional can generally
137   choose to use or prescribe an approved or cleared medical product for an unapproved use, if the
138   off-label use is appropriate based on his or her judgment. The narrow "safe harbor"
139   recommended in the guidance was also consistent with FDA's continued belief that FDA
140   premarket review and approval are critical to public health.
141

142   FDA is revising its 2009 guidance on good reprint practices in response to stakeholder questions
143   about its application to scientific and medical reference texts and CPGs that include or may
144   include[23] information on unapproved uses. This draft guidance provides recommendations for
145   scientific journal articles, scientific or medical reference texts, and CPGs in separate sections,
146   tailored to each type of publication. Consistent with longstanding FDA policy and practice, if
147   manufacturers distribute scientific or medical publications as recommended in this guidance,
148   FDA does not intend to use such distribution as evidence of the manufacturer's intent that the
149   product be used for an unapproved new use.
150

151   Although this draft guidance, like the 2009 guidance, recognizes the value to health care
152   professionals of truthful and non-misleading scientific or medical publications on unapproved
153   new uses, it also continues to recognize that this information is in no way a substitute for the

---

[22] For example, such information might be included as part of a manufacturer's response to an unsolicited request for off-label information. FDA has developed separate draft guidance that addresses how manufacturers can respond to unsolicited requests for off-label information related to their FDA-approved or -cleared products without such responses being used as evidence of intended use. See the draft guidance *Responding to Unsolicited Requests for Off-Label Information About Prescription Drugs and Medical Devices*, December 2011 (available at http://www.fda.gov/Drugs/GuidanceComplianceRegulatoryInformation/Guidances/default.htm). Once finalized, that draft guidance will represent the Agency's current thinking on this topic.

[23] For further explanation, see footnotes 31 and 39.

154 FDA premarket review process, which allows FDA to be proactive, rather than reactive, in
155 protecting the public from unsafe or ineffective medical products.
156
157 FDA is issuing this revised draft guidance to enable the public to provide comments on the
158 proposed approach.
159
160 **III.   RECOMMENDED PRACTICES**
161
162 Often scientific and medical information concerning the safety or effectiveness of a medical
163 product's unapproved new use may be published in scientific or medical journal articles,
164 scientific or medical reference texts, and/or in CPGs. These publications are available from their
165 publishers or other distribution channels, but have also been commonly distributed by
166 manufacturers to health care professionals and health care entities.
167
168 Sections A, B, and C, below, provide specific guidance for scientific and medical journal
169 articles, scientific and medical reference texts, and CPGs, respectively. FDA recommends that
170 manufacturers employ the following practices if they choose to disseminate scientific and
171 medical publications that include or may include information on unapproved new uses of
172 approved, cleared, or 510(k) exempt products.
173
174 **A.   Scientific or Medical Journal Articles**
175
176 If a manufacturer who chooses to distribute scientific or medical journal articles that include
177 information on unapproved/uncleared uses of its product(s) does so in accordance with the
178 recommendations of this guidance, FDA does not intend to use that distribution as evidence of
179 the manufacturer's intent that the product(s) be used for an unapproved new use.
180
181 A scientific or medical journal article that includes information on unapproved uses and is
182 distributed by manufacturers should first have been published by an organization that has an
183 editorial board that uses experts who have demonstrated expertise in the subject of the article
184 under review by the organization. Experts should be independent of the organization and should
185 review and objectively select, reject, or provide comments about proposed articles. Also, the
186 organization should adhere to a publicly stated policy of full disclosure of any conflict of interest
187 or biases for all authors, contributors, or editors associated with the journal or organization.
188
189 Additionally, the scientific or medical journal article distributed by a manufacturer *should*:
190
191   1. Be peer-reviewed and published in accordance with the peer-review procedures of the
192   organization.
193
194   2. Be in the form of an unabridged reprint or copy of an article.
195
196   3. Contain information that describes and addresses adequate and well-controlled clinical
197   investigations that are considered scientifically sound by experts with scientific training
198   and experience to evaluate the safety or effectiveness of the drug or device. In the case of
199   devices, significant investigations other than adequate and well-controlled studies, such

200 as meta-analyses, if they are testing a specific clinical hypothesis, and journal articles
201 discussing significant non-clinical research (such as well-designed bench or animal
202 studies) may be consistent with this guidance.
203
204   4. Be disseminated with the approved labeling or, in the case of a medical device reviewed
205   under section 510(k) of the FD&C Act (21 U.S.C. 360(k)), labeling for the indications in
206   the product's cleared indications for use statement, for each of the manufacturer's
207   products that is included in the distributed article.
208
209   5. Be disseminated with a comprehensive bibliography, when such information exists, of
210   publications discussing adequate and well-controlled clinical studies published in
211   scientific journals, medical journals, or scientific texts about the use of the drug or
212   medical device covered by the information disseminated (unless the information already
213   includes such a bibliography).
214
215   6. Be disseminated with a representative publication, when such information exists, that
216   reaches contrary or different conclusions regarding the unapproved use—especially when
217   the conclusions of articles to be disseminated have been specifically called into question
218   by another publication.
219
220   7. Be distributed separately from the delivery of information that is promotional in nature.
221   For example, if a sales representative delivers a reprint to a physician in his or her office,
222   the reprint should not be attached to any promotional material the sales representative
223   uses or delivers during the office visit. To the extent that the recipients of the scientific
224   or medical journal article have questions, the sales representative should refer the
225   questions to a medical/scientific officer or department, and the officer or department to
226   which the referral is made should be independent of the sales and/or marketing
227   departments. Similarly, while reprints may be distributed at medical or scientific
228   conferences in settings appropriate for scientific exchange, reprints should not be
229   distributed in promotional exhibit halls or during promotional speakers' programs.
230
231 A scientific or medical journal article that explains a use of a manufacturer's product and is
232 distributed by, or on behalf of, that manufacturer *must not:*
233
234   1. Be false or misleading.[24] For example, a distributed journal article should not be
235   characterized as definitive or representative of the weight of credible evidence derived
236   from adequate and well-controlled clinical investigations if it is inconsistent with the
237   weight of credible evidence or if a significant number of other studies contradict the
238   conclusions set forth in the article; should not have been withdrawn by the journal or
239   disclaimed by the author; and should not discuss a clinical investigation that FDA has
240   previously informed the company is not adequate and well-controlled.
241
242   2. Contain information recommending or suggesting use of the product that makes the
243   product dangerous to health when used in the manner suggested.[25]

---

[24] *See* sections 502(a), 201(m) of the FD&C Act. (21 U.S.C. 352(a), 321(m)).
[25] *See* sections 502(j), 201(m) of the FD&C Act. (21 U.S.C. 352(j), 321(m)).

244
245 To be consistent with the recommended practices described in this guidance, a scientific or
246 medical journal article regarding an unapproved use that is distributed by a manufacturer *should*
247 *not*:
248

1. Be in the form of a special supplement or publication that has been funded, in whole or in part, by one or more of the manufacturers of the product that is the subject of the article.

2. Be marked, highlighted, summarized, or characterized by the manufacturer, in writing or orally, to emphasize or promote an unapproved use. (This recommendation does not preclude providing the disclosures discussed elsewhere in this guidance.) For example, if during a sales call to a physician, a sales representative summarizes or characterizes the article to emphasize portions of the article that suggest the manufacturer's drug may be safe or effective for an unapproved use, this might be used as evidence of intended use.[26]

3. Be primarily distributed by a drug or device manufacturer; rather, it should be generally available in bookstores or other independent distribution channels (e.g., subscription, Internet) where periodicals are sold.

4. Be written, edited, excerpted, or published specifically for, or at the request of, a drug or device manufacturer.

5. Be edited or significantly influenced[27] by a drug or device manufacturer or any individuals having a financial relationship with the manufacturer.

6. Be attached to specific product information (other than the approved product labeling or the product's cleared indications for use statement).

The scientific or medical journal reprint *should be accompanied by* a prominently displayed and permanently affixed statement disclosing:

1. The drug(s) or device(s) included in the journal reprint in which the manufacturer has an interest.

2. That some or all uses of the manufacturer's drugs or devices described in the information have not been approved or cleared by FDA, as applicable to the described drug(s) or device(s).

---

[26] In addition, a distributed article must not be marked, highlighted, summarized, or characterized by the manufacturer in a manner that renders it false or misleading. See sections 502(a), 201(m) of the FD&C Act. (21 U.S.C. 352(a), 321(m)).

[27] FDA considers many factors when assessing whether a manufacturer is exercising significant influence over something or someone. For example, FDA examines the extent of control exercised by a manufacturer in a given scenario. See the FDA guidance for industry, *Industry-Supported Scientific and Educational Activities* (62 FR 64094, December 3, 1997), available at http://www.fda.gov/downloads/Drugs/GuidanceComplianceRegulatoryInformation/Guidances/ucm070072.pdf, for more examples of when something or someone may be considered to be independent from the significant influence of a firm.

281

282 3. Any author known to the manufacturer as having a financial interest in the manufacturer
283   or in a product of the manufacturer that is included in the journal article, or who is
284   receiving compensation from the manufacturer, along with the affiliation of the author, to
285   the extent known by the manufacturer, and the nature and amount of any such financial
286   interest of the author or compensation received by the author from the manufacturer.[28]

287

288 4. Any person known to the manufacturer who has provided funding for the study.

289

290 5. All significant risks or safety concerns associated with the unapproved use(s) of the
291   manufacturer's product(s) discussed in the journal article that are known to the
292   manufacturer but not discussed in the article.

293

294 The following types of journal reprints are examples that *would not* be considered consistent
295 with the recommended practices outlined in this guidance:

296

297 • Letters to the editor
298 • Abstracts of a publication
299 • Reports of healthy volunteer studies
300 • Publications consisting of statements or conclusions but which contain little or no
301   substantive discussion of the relevant investigation or data on which they are based

302

303 **B.   Scientific or Medical Reference Texts**

304

305 Scientific or medical reference texts[29] typically discuss a wide range of topics (e.g., medical
306 diagnosis, pathophysiology and treatments, pharmacology, surgical techniques, and other
307 scientific or medical information).[30] Like journal articles, scientific or medical reference texts
308 often contain information about unapproved use(s) of drugs and devices. However, because
309 these reference texts are considerably longer than journal articles, and generally address a wide
310 range of topics, FDA believes that it is appropriate to make specific recommendations for
311 distribution of reference texts that differ somewhat from the recommendations for journal
312 articles. If a manufacturer who chooses to distribute reference texts that include information on
313 unapproved/uncleared uses of its product(s) does so in accordance with the recommendations of
314 this guidance, FDA does not intend to use that distribution as evidence of the manufacturer's
315 intent that the product(s) be used for an unapproved new use.

316

317 A scientific or medical reference text that is distributed in its entirety by a manufacturer *should:*

318

---

[28] For purposes of this guidance, an *author* includes any individual, whether credited in the publication or not, who meets the standards for authorship set forth in the guidelines of the International Committee of Medical Journal Editors (available at http://www.icmje.org/recommendations/browse/roles-and-responsibilities/).

[29] For purposes of this guidance, there is no distinction between scientific and medical reference texts. Therefore, the recommendations presented here apply equally to both.

[30] FDA recognizes that certain scientific or medical reference texts address more specialized topics. The recommendations of this guidance also apply to distribution of these more specialized scientific or medical reference texts.

319   1. Be based on a systematic review of the existing evidence.
320
321   2. Be published (in print or electronic format) by an independent publisher, not substantially
322   dependent on financial support from drug or medical device manufacturers, who
323   publishes scientific or medical educational content for health care professionals and
324   students.
325
326   3. Be the most current version.
327
328   4. Be authored, edited, and/or contributed to by experts who have demonstrated expertise in
329   the subject area.
330
331   5. Be peer-reviewed by experts with relevant medical or scientific expertise and published
332   in accordance with the scientific or medical reference text peer-review procedures of the
333   publisher, which should be easily accessible or available upon request.
334
335   6. Be sold through usual and customary independent distribution channels (e.g., booksellers,
336   subscription, Internet) for medical and scientific educational content directed at health
337   care professionals and students.
338
339   7. Be distributed separately from the delivery of information that is promotional in nature.
340   For example, if a sales representative delivers a reference text (including individual
341   chapters) to a physician in his or her office, the reference text or chapter(s) should not be
342   attached to any promotional material the sales representative uses or delivers during the
343   office visit. To the extent that the recipients of scientific or medical reference texts have
344   questions, the sales representative should refer the questions to a medical/scientific
345   officer or department, and the officer or department to which the referral is made should
346   be independent of the sales and/or marketing departments. Similarly, while scientific or
347   medical reference texts may be distributed at medical or scientific conferences in settings
348   appropriate for scientific exchange, they should not be distributed in promotional exhibit
349   halls or during promotional speakers' programs.
350
351   8. Contain a prominently displayed and permanently affixed statement identifying the
352   distributing manufacturer and disclosing that some of the uses for drugs and/or devices
353   described in the reference text might not be approved or cleared by FDA. The statement
354   should also disclose that the author(s) of some chapters also might have a financial
355   interest in the manufacturer or its products, unless the manufacturer has verified that none
356   of the authors for the reference text has a financial interest in the manufacturer or a
357   product being written about.[31] This statement should be placed by sticker, stamp, or
358   other similar means on the front cover of the textbook.
359

---

[31] If a reference text is distributed in its entirety with this statement affixed, manufacturers are not expected to have reviewed every element of the reference text to identify discussions of off-label uses of their products. However, even where an entire reference text is being distributed, manufacturers should determine whether one or more individual chapters of that reference text devote primary substantive discussion to an individual product or products of the manufacturer distributing it, in order to determine whether dissemination of product labeling is recommended.

360   9.   In situations where a reference text is distributed in its entirety but one or more individual
361   chapters of that reference text devote primary substantive discussion to an individual
362   product or products of the manufacturer distributing it, be disseminated with the
363   approved product labeling for each such product or, in the case of a medical device
364   reviewed under section 510(k) of the FD&C Act (21 U.S.C. 360(k)), labeling for the
365   indications in the product's cleared indications for use statement.
366

367 If, in lieu of an entire scientific or medical reference text, a manufacturer distributes an
368 individual chapter(s) that includes information on unapproved/uncleared uses of the
369 manufacturer's product(s), the chapter(s) *should:*
370

371   1.   Come from a scientific or medical reference text that follows the recommendations for
372   complete scientific or medical reference texts in this guidance, except that the individual
373   chapter(s) should bear the prominently displayed and permanently affixed statement
374   described below for use on individual chapters, rather than the recommended statement
375   for texts distributed in their entirety.
376

377   2.   Be unaltered/unabridged and extracted directly from the scientific or medical reference
378   text in which it appears.
379

380   3.   When necessary to provide context, be disseminated with other unaltered/unabridged
381   chapters extracted directly from the same scientific or medical reference text, such as
382   chapters which provide related or supportive information.
383

384   4.   Contain a prominently displayed and permanently affixed statement identifying the
385   distributing manufacturer and disclosing:
386

387   (a) The drug(s) or device(s) addressed in the individual chapter(s) in which the
388   manufacturer has an interest;
389

390   (b) That some or all uses of the manufacturer's drugs and/or devices described in the
391   attached information have not been approved or cleared by FDA, as applicable to the
392   described drug(s) or medical device(s);
393

394   (c) Any author known to the manufacturer as having a financial interest in the
395   manufacturer or in a product of the manufacturer that is included in the individual
396   chapter(s), or who is receiving compensation from the manufacturer, along with the
397   affiliation of the author, to the extent known by the manufacturer, and the nature and
398   amount of any such financial interest of the author or compensation received by the
399   author from the manufacturer;
400

401   (d) All significant risks or safety concerns associated with the unapproved use(s) of the
402   manufacturer's products discussed in the individual chapter(s) that are known to the
403   manufacturer but not discussed in the chapter(s).
404

405   This statement should be placed by sticker, stamp, or other similar means on the front
406   page of each chapter.
407
408   5. Be disseminated with the approved labeling, or, in the case of a medical device reviewed
409   under section 510(k) of the FD&C Act (21 U.S.C. 360(k)), labeling for the indications in
410   the cleared indications for use statement, for each of the manufacturer's products that is
411   included in the distributed chapter(s).
412
413 A scientific or medical reference text, or an individual chapter, that explains a use of a
414 manufacturer's product and is distributed by, or on behalf of, that manufacturer *must not*:
415
416   1. Be false or misleading.[32]
417
418   2. Contain information recommending or suggesting use of the product in ways that make
419   the product dangerous to health when used in the manner suggested therein.[33]
420
421 To be consistent with the recommended practices described in this guidance, a scientific or
422 medical reference text, or an individual chapter, that is distributed *should not*:
423
424   1. Be primarily distributed by a drug or device manufacturer; rather, it should be generally
425   available in bookstores or other independent distribution channels (e.g., subscription,
426   Internet) where textbooks are sold.
427
428   2. Be edited or significantly influenced by a drug or device manufacturer or any individuals
429   having a financial relationship with the manufacturer.
430
431   3. Be marked, highlighted, summarized, or characterized by the manufacturer, in writing or
432   orally, to emphasize or promote an unapproved use. (This recommendation does not
433   preclude providing the disclosures discussed elsewhere in this guidance.) For example, if
434   during a sales call to a physician, a sales representative summarizes or characterizes the
435   text to emphasize passages that suggest that a drug of the manufacturer may be safe or
436   effective for an unapproved use, this might be used as evidence of intended use.[34]
437
438   4. Be written or published specifically at the request of a drug or device manufacturer.
439
440   5. Be abridged or excerpted[35] in any particular manner.
441

---

[32] *See* sections 502(a), 201(m) of the FD&C Act. (21 U.S.C. 352(a), 321(m)).

[33] *See* sections 502(j), 201(m) of the FD&C Act. (21 U.S.C. 352(j), 321(m)).

[34] In addition, a distributed reference text must not be marked, highlighted, summarized, or characterized by the manufacturer in a manner that renders it false or misleading. See sections 502(a), 201(m) of the FD&C Act. (21 U.S.C. 352(a), 321(m)).

[35] In situations where the entire reference text is being disseminated, the reference text should be complete and no chapters excerpted in any manner. In situations where individual chapters of a reference text are being disseminated, the individual chapters should be complete. In other words, an excerpt from an individual chapter would not satisfy the recommendations outlined in this guidance pertaining to the dissemination of individual chapters of scientific or medical reference texts.

442   6. Be attached to specific product information (other than the approved product labeling or
443   the product's cleared indications for use statement).
444

445   **C.   Clinical Practice Guidelines**
446

447   CPGs are statements that include recommendations intended to help clinicians make decisions
448   for individual patient care, including in circumstances where there are few or no approved drugs
449   or devices indicated for the patient's condition or the approved therapies have not proven
450   successful for the individual. A CPG may be much longer and often covers a wider range of
451   topics than a journal article. FDA believes that it is appropriate to make specific
452   recommendations for manufacturer distribution of CPGs that include information on unapproved
453   new uses of that manufacturer's approved or cleared products that differ somewhat from the
454   recommendations for journal articles. These recommendations are set forth below, along with
455   additional recommendations that incorporate the Institute of Medicine's (IOM's) standards for
456   CPG "trustworthiness."[36] These "trustworthiness" standards, among other things, ensure that
457   CPGs are informed by a systematic review of evidence and an assessment of the benefits and
458   harms of alternative care options.
459

460   If a manufacturer who chooses to distribute CPGs that include information on
461   unapproved/uncleared uses of its product(s) does so in accordance with the recommendations of
462   this guidance, FDA does not intend to use that distribution as evidence of the manufacturer's
463   intent that the product(s) be used for an unapproved new use.
464

465   Drug and medical device manufacturers wishing to disseminate CPGs that discuss unapproved or
466   uncleared new uses of products that they market should disseminate only those guidelines that
467   are "trustworthy," as described below. In keeping with the IOM standards, to be considered
468   "trustworthy," a CPG *should* at minimum:
469

470   1. Be based on a systematic review of the existing evidence.
471

472   2. Be developed by a knowledgeable, multidisciplinary panel of experts and representatives
473   from key affected groups.
474

475   3. Consider important patient subgroups and patient preferences.
476

---

[36] Through the Medicare Improvements for Patients and Providers Act of 2008, Congress required the Secretary of Health and Human Services (HHS) to contract with IOM (through the Agency for Healthcare Research and Quality (AHRQ)) to undertake a study that focused on "the best methods used in developing clinical practice guidelines in order to ensure that organizations developing such guidelines have information on approaches that are objective, scientifically valid, and consistent." Pub. L. No. 110-275, 122 Stat. 2595. Also, in this legislation, Congress required IOM to submit a report to the Secretary of HHS and the appropriate committees of Congress containing the results of the study, together with recommendations for such legislation and administrative action as IOM determines appropriate. The standards for CPG "trustworthiness," as incorporated in this guidance, are taken directly from IOM's study results (as articulated in its report, Robin Graham, et al., Institute of Medicine of the National Academies, Committee on Standards for Developing Trustworthy Clinical Practice Guidelines, *Clinical Practice Guidelines We Can Trust* (2011)).

477   4. Be based on an explicit and transparent (publicly accessible) process by which the CPG is
478   developed and funded that minimizes distortions,[37] biases, and conflicts of interest.
479

480   5. Provide a clear explanation of the logical relationships between alternative care options
481   and health outcomes, provide clearly articulated recommendations in standardized form,
482   and provide ratings of both quality of evidence and the strength of recommendations.
483

484   6. Be reconsidered and revised when important new evidence warrants modifications of
485   recommendations.[38]
486

487 Manufacturers wishing to distribute a "trustworthy" CPG in its entirety *should*:
488

489   1. Ensure that the most current version of the CPG is disseminated.
490

491   2. Distribute the CPG separately from the delivery of information that is promotional in
492   nature. For example, if a sales representative delivers a CPG to a physician in his or her
493   office, the CPG should not be attached to any promotional material the sales
494   representative uses or delivers during the office visit. To the extent that the recipients of
495   the CPG have questions, the sales representative should refer the questions to a
496   medical/scientific officer or department, and the officer or department to which the
497   referral is made should be independent of the sales and/or marketing departments.
498   Similarly, while a CPG may be distributed at medical or scientific conferences in settings
499   appropriate for scientific exchange, the CPG should not be distributed in promotional
500   exhibit halls or during promotional speakers' programs.
501

502   3. Ensure that the CPG contains a prominently displayed and permanently affixed statement
503   identifying the distributing manufacturer and disclosing that some of the uses of drugs
504   and/or devices described in the CPG might not be approved or cleared by FDA. The
505   statement should also disclose that the author(s) of some sections might have a financial
506   interest in the manufacturer or its products, unless the manufacturer has verified that none
507   of the authors for the CPG has a financial interest in the manufacturer or a product being
508   written about. This statement should be placed by sticker, stamp, or other similar means
509   on the front page of the CPG.[39]
510

511   4. In situations where a CPG is distributed in its entirety but one or more individual sections
512   of that CPG devotes primary substantive discussion to an individual product or products
513   of the manufacturer distributing it, be disseminated with the approved product labeling
514   for each such product or, in the case of a medical device reviewed under section 510(k)

---

[37] Distortion may result from, for example, reliance on incomplete data.

[38] For a more in-depth discussion of the standards, including any adherence concerns, please see the IOM report referenced in footnote 36, available at http://www.iom.edu/Reports/2011/Clinical-Practice-Guidelines-We-Can-Trust.aspx.

[39] If a CPG is distributed in its entirety with this statement affixed, manufacturers are not expected to have reviewed every element of the CPG to identify discussions of off-label uses of their products. However, even where an entire CPG is being distributed, manufacturers should determine whether one or more individual sections of that CPG devote primary substantive discussion to an individual product or products of the manufacturer distributing it, in order to determine whether dissemination of product labeling is recommended.

of the FD&C Act (21 U.S.C. 360(k)), labeling for the indications in the product's cleared indications for use statement.

If, in lieu of an entire CPG, a manufacturer distributes an individual section(s) that includes information on unapproved/uncleared uses of the manufacturer's product(s),[40] the section(s) *should:*

1. Come from a CPG that satisfies the recommendations set forth in this guidance, including the standards for "trustworthiness," except that the section should bear the prominently displayed and permanently affixed statement described below for use on individual sections, rather than the recommended statement for CPGs distributed in their entirety.

2. Be unaltered/unabridged and extracted directly from the CPG in which it appears.

3. When necessary to provide context, be disseminated with other unaltered/unabridged sections extracted directly from the same CPG, such as sections which provide related or supportive information.

4. Contain a prominently displayed and permanently affixed statement identifying the distributing manufacturer and disclosing:

    (a) The drug(s) or device(s) addressed in the individual section(s) in which the manufacturer has an interest;

    (b) That some or all uses of the manufacturer's drugs and/or devices described in the attached information have not been approved or cleared by FDA, as applicable to the described drug(s) or medical device(s);

    (c) Any author known to the manufacturer as having a financial interest in the manufacturer or in a product of the manufacturer that is included in the individual section(s), or who is receiving compensation from the manufacturer, along with the affiliation of the author, to the extent known by the manufacturer, and the nature and amount of any such financial interest of the author or compensation received by the author from the manufacturer;

    (d) All significant risks or safety concerns associated with the unapproved use(s) of the manufacturer's products discussed in the individual section(s) that are known to the manufacturer but not discussed in the section(s).

    This statement should be placed by sticker, stamp, or other similar means on the front page of each section.

---

[40] A CPG that addresses only one disease state should be disseminated in its entirety. If a CPG substantively addresses multiple disease states, and manufacturers wish to disseminate only certain sections of the CPG, they should follow the recommendations discussed below.

557 5. Be disseminated with the approved labeling, or, in the case of a medical device reviewed
558 under section 510(k) of the FD&C Act (21 U.S.C. 360(k)), labeling for the indications in
559 the cleared indications for use statement, for each of the manufacturer's products that is
560 included in the distributed section(s).

561

562 A CPG or individual section(s) of a CPG that explains a use of a manufacturer's product and is
563 distributed by, or on behalf of, that manufacturer *must not:*

564

565 1. Be false or misleading.[41]

566

567 2. Contain information recommending or suggesting use of the product in ways that make
568 the product dangerous to health when used in the manner suggested therein.[42]

569

570 To be consistent with the recommended practices described in this guidance, a CPG or individual
571 section of a CPG that discusses unapproved new uses of a manufacturer's product *should not:*

572

573 1. Be primarily distributed by a drug or device manufacturer, but should be generally
574 available through other independent distribution channels (e.g., subscription, Internet).

575

576 2. Be edited or significantly influenced[43] by a drug or device manufacturer or any
577 individuals having a financial relationship with the manufacturer.

578

579 3. Be marked, highlighted, summarized, or characterized by the manufacturer in writing or
580 orally, to emphasize or promote an unapproved use. (This recommendation does not
581 preclude providing the disclosures discussed elsewhere in this guidance.) For example, if
582 during a sales call to a physician, a sales representative summarizes or characterizes the
583 CPG to emphasize portions that suggest the manufacturer's product may be safe or
584 effective for an unapproved use, this might be used as evidence of intended use.[44]

585

586 4. Be written or published specifically at the request of a drug or device manufacturer.

587

588 5. Be abridged or excerpted[45] in any particular manner.

589

590 6. Be attached to specific product information (other than the approved product labeling or
591 the product's cleared indications for use statement).

---

[41] *See* sections 502(a), 201(m) of the FD&C Act. (21 U.S.C. 352(a), 321(m)).

[42] *See* sections 502(j), 201(m) of the FD&C Act. (21 U.S.C. 352(j), 321(m)).

[43] Please see footnote 27 for further information regarding FDA's understanding of "significant influence."

[44] In addition, a distributed CPG must not be marked, highlighted, summarized, or characterized by the manufacturer in a manner that renders it false or misleading. See sections 502(a), 201(m) of the FD&C Act. (21 U.S.C. 352(a), 321(m)).

[45] In situations where an entire CPG is being disseminated, the CPG should be complete and no sections excerpted in any manner. In situations where individual sections of a CPG are being disseminated, the individual sections should be complete. In other words, an excerpt from an individual section would not satisfy the recommendations outlined in this guidance pertaining to the dissemination of individual sections of a CPG.

FOOD AND DRUG ADMINISTRATION
MODERIZATION ACT OF 1997

PUBLIC LAW 105–115—NOV. 21, 1997

Public Law 105–115
105th Congress

An Act

Nov. 21, 1997
[S. 830]

To amend the Federal Food, Drug, and Cosmetic Act and the Public Health Service Act to improve the regulation of food, drugs, devices, and biological products, and for other purposes.

Be it enacted by the Senate and House of Representatives of the United States of America in Congress assembled,

Food and Drug Administration Modernization Act of 1997.

21 USC 301 note.

SECTION 1. SHORT TITLE; REFERENCES; TABLE OF CONTENTS.

(a) SHORT TITLE.—This Act may be cited as the "Food and Drug Administration Modernization Act of 1997".

(b) REFERENCES.—Except as otherwise specified, whenever in this Act an amendment or repeal is expressed in terms of an amendment to or a repeal of a section or other provision, the reference shall be considered to be made to that section or other provision of the Federal Food, Drug, and Cosmetic Act (21 U.S.C. 301 et seq.).

(c) TABLE OF CONTENTS.—The table of contents for this Act is as follows:

SEC. 2. DEFINITIONS.   21 USC 321 note.

In this Act, the terms "drug", "device", "food", and "dietary supplement" have the meaning given such terms in section 201 of the Federal Food, Drug, and Cosmetic Act (21 U.S.C. 321).

TITLE I—IMPROVING REGULATION OF DRUGS

Subtitle A—Fees Relating to Drugs

21 USC 379g note.

SEC. 101. FINDINGS.

Congress finds that—

(1) prompt approval of safe and effective new drugs and other therapies is critical to the improvement of the public health so that patients may enjoy the benefits provided by these therapies to treat and prevent illness and disease;

(2) the public health will be served by making additional funds available for the purpose of augmenting the resources of the Food and Drug Administration that are devoted to the process for review of human drug applications;

(3) the provisions added by the Prescription Drug User Fee Act of 1992 have been successful in substantially reducing review times for human drug applications and should be—

(A) reauthorized for an additional 5 years, with certain technical improvements; and

(B) carried out by the Food and Drug Administration with new commitments to implement more ambitious and comprehensive improvements in regulatory processes of the Food and Drug Administration; and

(4) the fees authorized by amendments made in this subtitle will be dedicated toward expediting the drug development process and the review of human drug applications as set forth in the goals identified, for purposes of part 2 of subchapter C of chapter VII of the Federal Food, Drug, and Cosmetic Act, in the letters from the Secretary of Health and Human Services to the chairman of the Committee on Commerce of the House of Representatives and the chairman of the Committee on Labor and Human Resources of the Senate, as set forth in the Congressional Record.

SEC. 102. DEFINITIONS.

Section 735 (21 U.S.C. 379g) is amended—

(1) in the second sentence of paragraph (1)—

(A) by striking "Service Act, and" and inserting "Service Act,"; and

(B) by striking "September 1, 1992." and inserting the following: "September 1, 1992, does not include an application for a licensure of a biological product for further manufacturing use only, and does not include an application or supplement submitted by a State or Federal Government entity for a drug that is not distributed commercially. Such term does include an application for licensure, as described in subparagraph (D), of a large volume biological product intended for single dose injection for intravenous use or infusion.";

(2) in the second sentence of paragraph (3)—

(A) by striking "Service Act, and" and inserting "Service Act,"; and

(B) by striking "September 1, 1992." and inserting the following: "September 1, 1992, does not include a biological product that is licensed for further manufacturing use only, and does not include a drug that is not distributed commercially and is the subject of an application or supplement submitted by a State or Federal Government entity. Such term does include a large volume biological product intended for single dose injection for intravenous use or infusion.";

(3) in paragraph (4), by striking "without" and inserting "without substantial";

(4) by amending the first sentence of paragraph (5) to read as follows:

"(5) The term 'prescription drug establishment' means a foreign or domestic place of business which is at one general physical location consisting of one or more buildings all of which are within five miles of each other and at which one or more prescription drug products are manufactured in final dosage form.";

(5) in paragraph (7)(A)—

(A) by striking "employees under contract" and all that follows through "Administration," the second time it occurs and inserting "contractors of the Food and Drug Administration,"; and

(B) by striking "and committees," and inserting "and committees and to contracts with such contractors,";

(6) in paragraph (8)—

(A) in subparagraph (A)—

(i) by striking "August of" and inserting "April of"; and

(ii) by striking "August 1992" and inserting "April 1997"; and

(B) in subparagraph (B)—

(i) by striking "section 254(d)" and inserting "section 254(c)";

(ii) by striking "1992" and inserting "1997"; and

(iii) by striking "102d Congress, 2d Session" and inserting "105th Congress, 1st Session"; and

(7) by adding at the end the following:

"(9) The term 'affiliate' means a business entity that has a relationship with a second business entity if, directly or indirectly—

"(A) one business entity controls, or has the power to control, the other business entity; or

"(B) a third party controls, or has power to control, both of the business entities.".

SEC. 103. AUTHORITY TO ASSESS AND USE DRUG FEES.

(a) TYPES OF FEES.—Section 736(a) (21 U.S.C. 379h(a)) is amended—

(1) by striking "Beginning in fiscal year 1993" and inserting "Beginning in fiscal year 1998";

(2) in paragraph (1)—

(A) by striking subparagraph (B) and inserting the following:

"(B) PAYMENT.—The fee required by subparagraph (A) shall be due upon submission of the application or supplement.";

(B) in subparagraph (D)—

(i) in the subparagraph heading, by striking "NOT ACCEPTED" and inserting "REFUSED";

(ii) by striking "50 percent" and inserting "75 percent";

(iii) by striking "subparagraph (B)(i)" and inserting "subparagraph (B)"; and

(iv) by striking "not accepted" and inserting "refused"; and

(C) by adding at the end the following:

"(E) EXCEPTION FOR DESIGNATED ORPHAN DRUG OR INDICATION.—A human drug application for a prescription drug product that has been designated as a drug for a rare disease or condition pursuant to section 526 shall not be subject to a fee under subparagraph (A), unless the human drug application includes an indication for other than a rare disease or condition. A supplement proposing to include a new indication for a rare disease or condition in a human drug application shall not be subject to a fee under subparagraph (A), if the drug has been designated pursuant to section 526 as a drug for a rare disease or condition with regard to the indication proposed in such supplement.

"(F) EXCEPTION FOR SUPPLEMENTS FOR PEDIATRIC INDICATIONS.—A supplement to a human drug application proposing to include a new indication for use in pediatric populations shall not be assessed a fee under subparagraph (A).

"(G) REFUND OF FEE IF APPLICATION WITHDRAWN.— If an application or supplement is withdrawn after the application or supplement was filed, the Secretary may refund the fee or a portion of the fee if no substantial work was performed on the application or supplement after the application or supplement was filed. The Secretary shall have the sole discretion to refund a fee or a portion of the fee under this subparagraph. A determination by the Secretary concerning a refund under this paragraph shall not be reviewable.";

(3) by striking paragraph (2) and inserting the following:

"(2) PRESCRIPTION DRUG ESTABLISHMENT FEE.—

"(A) IN GENERAL.—Except as provided in subparagraph (B), each person that—

"(i) is named as the applicant in a human drug application; and

"(ii) after September 1, 1992, had pending before the Secretary a human drug application or supplement, shall be assessed an annual fee established in subsection (b) for each prescription drug establishment listed in its approved human drug application as an establishment that manufactures the prescription drug product named in the application. The annual establishment fee shall be assessed in each fiscal year in which the prescription drug product named in the application is assessed a fee under paragraph (3) unless the prescription drug establishment listed in the application does not engage in the manufacture of the prescription drug product during the fiscal year. The establishment fee shall be payable on or before January 31 of each year. Each such establishment shall be assessed only one fee per establishment, notwithstanding the number of prescription drug products manufactured at the establishment. In the event an establishment is listed in a human drug application by more than one applicant, the establishment fee for the fiscal year shall be divided equally and assessed among the applicants whose prescription drug products are manufactured by the establishment during the fiscal year and assessed product fees under paragraph (3).

"(B) EXCEPTION.—If, during the fiscal year, an applicant initiates or causes to be initiated the manufacture of a prescription drug product at an establishment listed in its human drug application—

"(i) that did not manufacture the product in the previous fiscal year; and

"(ii) for which the full establishment fee has been assessed in the fiscal year at a time before manufacture of the prescription drug product was begun;

the applicant will not be assessed a share of the establishment fee for the fiscal year in which the manufacture of the product began."; and

(4) in paragraph (3)—

(A) in subparagraph (A)—

(i) in clause (i), by striking "is listed" and inserting "has been submitted for listing"; and

(ii) by striking "Such fee shall be payable" and all that follows through "section 510." and inserting the following: "Such fee shall be payable for the fiscal year in which the product is first submitted for listing under section 510, or is submitted for relisting under section 510 if the product has been withdrawn from listing and relisted. After such fee is paid for that fiscal year, such fee shall be payable on or before January 31 of each year. Such fee shall be paid only once for each product for a fiscal year in which the fee is payable."; and

(B) in subparagraph (B), by striking "505(j)." and inserting the following: "505(j), under an abbreviated application filed under section 507 (as in effect on the day before the date of enactment of the Food and Drug Administration Modernization Act of 1997), or under an abbreviated new drug application pursuant to regulations in effect prior to the implementation of the Drug Price Competition and Patent Term Restoration Act of 1984.".

(b) FEE AMOUNTS.—Section 736(b) (21 U.S.C. 379h(b)) is amended to read as follows:

"(b) FEE AMOUNTS.—Except as provided in subsections (c), (d), (f), and (g), the fees required under subsection (a) shall be determined and assessed as follows:

"(1) APPLICATION AND SUPPLEMENT FEES.—

"(A) FULL FEES.—The application fee under subsection (a)(1)(A)(i) shall be $250,704 in fiscal year 1998, $256,338 in each of fiscal years 1999 and 2000, $267,606 in fiscal year 2001, and $258,451 in fiscal year 2002.

"(B) OTHER FEES.—The fee under subsection (a)(1)(A)(ii) shall be $125,352 in fiscal year 1998, $128,169 in each of fiscal years 1999 and 2000, $133,803 in fiscal year 2001, and $129,226 in fiscal year 2002.

"(2) TOTAL FEE REVENUES FOR ESTABLISHMENT FEES.—The total fee revenues to be collected in establishment fees under subsection (a)(2) shall be $35,600,000 in fiscal year 1998, $36,400,000 in each of fiscal years 1999 and 2000, $38,000,000 in fiscal year 2001, and $36,700,000 in fiscal year 2002.

"(3) TOTAL FEE REVENUES FOR PRODUCT FEES.—The total fee revenues to be collected in product fees under subsection (a)(3) in a fiscal year shall be equal to the total fee revenues collected in establishment fees under subsection (a)(2) in that fiscal year.".

(c) INCREASES AND ADJUSTMENTS.—Section 736(c) (21 U.S.C. 379h(c)) is amended—

(1) in the subsection heading, by striking "INCREASES AND";

(2) in paragraph (1)—

(A) by striking "(1) REVENUE" and all that follows through "increased by the Secretary" and inserting the following: "(1) INFLATION ADJUSTMENT.—The fees and total fee revenues established in subsection (b) shall be adjusted by the Secretary";

(B) in subparagraph (A), by striking "increase" and inserting "change";

(C) in subparagraph (B), by striking "increase" and inserting "change"; and

(D) by adding at the end the following flush sentence: "The adjustment made each fiscal year by this subsection will be added on a compounded basis to the sum of all adjustments made each fiscal year after fiscal year 1997 under this subsection.";

(3) in paragraph (2), by striking "October 1, 1992," and all that follows through "such schedule." and inserting the following: "September 30, 1997, adjust the establishment and product fees described in subsection (b) for the fiscal year in which the adjustment occurs so that the revenues collected from each of the categories of fees described in paragraphs (2) and (3) of subsection (b) shall be set to be equal to the revenues collected from the category of application and supplement fees described in paragraph (1) of subsection (b)."; and

(4) in paragraph (3), by striking "paragraph (2)" and inserting "this subsection".

(d) FEE WAIVER OR REDUCTION.—Section 736(d) (21 U.S.C. 379h(d)) is amended—

(1) by redesignating paragraphs (1), (2), (3), and (4) as subparagraphs (A), (B), (C), and (D), respectively and indenting appropriately;

(2) by striking "The Secretary shall grant a" and all that follows through "finds that—" and inserting the following: "(1) IN GENERAL.—The Secretary shall grant a waiver from or a reduction of one or more fees assessed under subsection (a) where the Secretary finds that—";

(3) in subparagraph (C) (as so redesignated in paragraph (1)), by striking ", or" and inserting a comma;

(4) in subparagraph (D) (as so redesignated in paragraph (1)), by striking the period and inserting ", or";

(5) by inserting after subparagraph (D) (as so redesignated in paragraph (1)) the following:

"(E) the applicant involved is a small business submitting its first human drug application to the Secretary for review."; and

(6) by striking "In making the finding in paragraph (3)," and all that follows through "standard costs." and inserting the following:

"(2) USE OF STANDARD COSTS.—In making the finding in paragraph (1)(C), the Secretary may use standard costs.

"(3) RULES RELATING TO SMALL BUSINESSES.—

"(A) DEFINITION.—In paragraph (1)(E), the term 'small business' means an entity that has fewer than 500 employees, including employees of affiliates.

"(B) WAIVER OF APPLICATION FEE.—The Secretary shall waive under paragraph (1)(E) the application fee for the first human drug application that a small business or its affiliate submits to the Secretary for review. After a small business or its affiliate is granted such a waiver, the small business or its affiliate shall pay—

"(i) application fees for all subsequent human drug applications submitted to the Secretary for review in the same manner as an entity that does not qualify as a small business; and

"(ii) all supplement fees for all supplements to human drug applications submitted to the Secretary for review in the same manner as an entity that does not qualify as a small business.".

(e) ASSESSMENT OF FEES.—Section 736(f)(1) (21 U.S.C. 379h(f)(1)) is amended—

(1) by striking "fiscal year 1993" and inserting "fiscal year 1997"; and

(2) by striking "fiscal year 1992" and inserting "fiscal year 1997 (excluding the amount of fees appropriated for such fiscal year)".

(f) CREDITING AND AVAILABILITY OF FEES.—Section 736(g) (21 U.S.C. 379h(g)) is amended—

(1) in paragraph (1), by adding at the end the following: "Such sums as may be necessary may be transferred from the Food and Drug Administration salaries and expenses appropriation account without fiscal year limitation to such appropriation account for salaries and expenses with such fiscal year limitation. The sums transferred shall be available solely for the process for the review of human drug applications.";

(2) in paragraph (2)—

(A) in subparagraph (A), by striking "Acts" and inserting "Acts, or otherwise made available for obligation,"; and

(B) in subparagraph (B), by striking "over such costs for fiscal year 1992" and inserting "over such costs, excluding costs paid from fees collected under this section, for fiscal year 1997"; and

(3) by striking paragraph (3) and inserting the following:

"(3) AUTHORIZATION OF APPROPRIATIONS.—There are authorized to be appropriated for fees under this section—

"(A) $106,800,000 for fiscal year 1998;

"(B) $109,200,000 for fiscal year 1999;

"(C) $109,200,000 for fiscal year 2000;

"(D) $114,000,000 for fiscal year 2001; and

"(E) $110,100,000 for fiscal year 2002,

as adjusted to reflect adjustments in the total fee revenues made under this section and changes in the total amounts collected by application, supplement, establishment, and product fees.

"(4) OFFSET.—Any amount of fees collected for a fiscal year under this section that exceeds the amount of fees specified in appropriation Acts for such fiscal year shall be credited to the appropriation account of the Food and Drug Administration as provided in paragraph (1), and shall be subtracted from the amount of fees that would otherwise be authorized to be collected under this section pursuant to appropriation Acts for a subsequent fiscal year.".

(g) REQUIREMENT FOR WRITTEN REQUESTS FOR WAIVERS, REDUCTIONS, AND REFUNDS.—Section 736 (21 U.S.C. 379h) is amended—

(1) by redesignating subsection (i) as subsection (j); and

(2) by inserting after subsection (h) the following:

"(i) WRITTEN REQUESTS FOR WAIVERS, REDUCTIONS, AND REFUNDS.—To qualify for consideration for a waiver or reduction under subsection (d), or for a refund of any fee collected in accordance with subsection (a), a person shall submit to the Secretary a written request for such waiver, reduction, or refund not later than 180 days after such fee is due.".

21 USC 379h note.

(h) SPECIAL RULE FOR WAIVERS AND REFUNDS.—Any requests for waivers or refunds for fees assessed under section 736 of the Federal Food, Drug, and Cosmetic Act (42 U.S.C. 379h) prior to the date of enactment of this Act shall be submitted in writing to the Secretary of Health and Human Services within 1 year after the date of enactment of this Act. Any requests for waivers or refunds pertaining to a fee for a human drug application or supplement accepted for filing prior to October 1, 1997 or to a product or establishment fee required by such Act for a fiscal year prior to fiscal year 1998, shall be evaluated according to the terms of the Prescription Drug User Fee Act of 1992 (as in effect on September 30, 1997) and part 2 of subchapter C of chapter VII of the Federal Food, Drug, and Cosmetic Act (as in effect on September 30, 1997). The term "person" in such Acts shall continue to include an affiliate thereof.

21 USC 379g note.

SEC. 104. ANNUAL REPORTS.

(a) PERFORMANCE REPORT.—Beginning with fiscal year 1998, not later than 60 days after the end of each fiscal year during which fees are collected under part 2 of subchapter C of chapter VII of the Federal Food, Drug, and Cosmetic Act (21 U.S.C. 379g et seq.), the Secretary of Health and Human Services shall prepare and submit to the Committee on Commerce of the House of Representatives and the Committee on Labor and Human Resources of the Senate a report concerning the progress of the Food and Drug Administration in achieving the goals identified in the letters described in section 101(4) during such fiscal year and the future plans of the Food and Drug Administration for meeting the goals.

(b) FISCAL REPORT.—Beginning with fiscal year 1998, not later than 120 days after the end of each fiscal year during which fees are collected under the part described in subsection (a), the Secretary of Health and Human Services shall prepare and submit to the Committee on Commerce of the House of Representatives and the Committee on Labor and Human Resources of the Senate a report on the implementation of the authority for such fees during such fiscal year and the use, by the Food and Drug Administration, of the fees collected during such fiscal year for which the report is made.

SEC. 105. SAVINGS.

21 USC 379g note.

Notwithstanding section 105 of the Prescription Drug User Fee Act of 1992, the Secretary shall retain the authority to assess and collect any fee required by part 2 of subchapter C of chapter VII of the Federal Food, Drug, and Cosmetic Act for a human drug application or supplement accepted for filing prior to October 1, 1997, and to assess and collect any product or establishment fee required by such Act for a fiscal year prior to fiscal year 1998.

SEC. 106. EFFECTIVE DATE.

21 USC 379g note.

The amendments made by this subtitle shall take effect October 1, 1997.

SEC. 107. TERMINATION OF EFFECTIVENESS.

21 USC 379g note.

The amendments made by sections 102 and 103 cease to be effective October 1, 2002, and section 104 ceases to be effective 120 days after such date.

Subtitle B—Other Improvements

SEC. 111. PEDIATRIC STUDIES OF DRUGS.

Chapter V (21 U.S.C. 351 et seq.) is amended by inserting after section 505 the following:

"SEC. 505A. PEDIATRIC STUDIES OF DRUGS.

21 USC 355a.

"(a) MARKET EXCLUSIVITY FOR NEW DRUGS.—If, prior to approval of an application that is submitted under section 505(b)(1), the Secretary determines that information relating to the use of a new drug in the pediatric population may produce health benefits in that population, the Secretary makes a written request for pediatric studies (which shall include a timeframe for completing such studies), and such studies are completed within any such timeframe and the reports thereof submitted in accordance with subsection (d)(2) or accepted in accordance with subsection (d)(3)—

"(1)(A)(i) the period referred to in subsection (c)(3)(D)(ii) of section 505, and in subsection (j)(4)(D)(ii) of such section, is deemed to be five years and six months rather than five years, and the references in subsections (c)(3)(D)(ii) and (j)(4)(D)(ii) of such section to four years, to forty-eight months, and to seven and one-half years are deemed to be four and one-half years, fifty-four months, and eight years, respectively; or

"(ii) the period referred to in clauses (iii) and (iv) of subsection (c)(3)(D) of such section, and in clauses (iii) and (iv) of subsection (j)(4)(D) of such section, is deemed to be three years and six months rather than three years; and

"(B) if the drug is designated under section 526 for a rare disease or condition, the period referred to in section 527(a) is deemed to be seven years and six months rather than seven years; and

"(2)(A) if the drug is the subject of—

"(i) a listed patent for which a certification has been submitted under subsection (b)(2)(A)(ii) or (j)(2)(A)(vii)(II) of section 505 and for which pediatric studies were submitted prior to the expiration of the patent (including any patent extensions); or

"(ii) a listed patent for which a certification has been submitted under subsections (b)(2)(A)(iii) or (j)(2)(A)(vii)(III) of section 505,

the period during which an application may not be approved under section 505(c)(3) or section 505(j)(4)(B) shall be extended by a period of six months after the date the patent expires (including any patent extensions); or

"(B) if the drug is the subject of a listed patent for which a certification has been submitted under subsection (b)(2)(A)(iv) or (j)(2)(A)(vii)(IV) of section 505, and in the patent infringement litigation resulting from the certification the court determines that the patent is valid and would be infringed, the period during which an application may not be approved under section 505(c)(3) or section 505(j)(4)(B) shall be extended by a period of six months after the date the patent expires (including any patent extensions).

"(b) SECRETARY TO DEVELOP LIST OF DRUGS FOR WHICH ADDITIONAL PEDIATRIC INFORMATION MAY BE BENEFICIAL.—Not later than 180 days after the date of enactment of the Food and Drug Administration Modernization Act of 1997, the Secretary, after consultation with experts in pediatric research shall develop, prioritize, and publish an initial list of approved drugs for which additional pediatric information may produce health benefits in the pediatric population. The Secretary shall annually update the list.

"(c) MARKET EXCLUSIVITY FOR ALREADY-MARKETED DRUGS.— If the Secretary makes a written request to the holder of an approved application under section 505(b)(1) for pediatric studies (which shall include a timeframe for completing such studies) concerning a drug identified in the list described in subsection (b), the holder agrees to the request, the studies are completed within any such timeframe, and the reports thereof are submitted in accordance with subsection (d)(2) or accepted in accordance with subsection (d)(3)—

"(1)(A)(i) the period referred to in subsection (c)(3)(D)(ii) of section 505, and in subsection (j)(4)(D)(ii) of such section, is deemed to be five years and six months rather than five years, and the references in subsections (c)(3)(D)(ii) and (j)(4)(D)(ii) of such section to four years, to forty-eight months, and to seven and one-half years are deemed to be four and one-half years, fifty-four months, and eight years, respectively; or

"(ii) the period referred to in clauses (iii) and (iv) of subsection (c)(3)(D) of such section, and in clauses (iii) and (iv) of subsection (j)(4)(D) of such section, is deemed to be three years and six months rather than three years; and

"(B) if the drug is designated under section 526 for a rare disease or condition, the period referred to in section 527(a) is deemed to be seven years and six months rather than seven years; and

"(2)(A) if the drug is the subject of—

"(i) a listed patent for which a certification has been submitted under subsection (b)(2)(A)(ii) or (j)(2)(A)(vii)(II) of section 505 and for which pediatric studies were submitted prior to the expiration of the patent (including any patent extensions); or

"(ii) a listed patent for which a certification has been submitted under subsection (b)(2)(A)(iii) or (j)(2)(A)(vii)(III) of section 505,

the period during which an application may not be approved under section 505(c)(3) or section 505(j)(4)(B) shall be extended by a period of six months after the date the patent expires (including any patent extensions); or

"(B) if the drug is the subject of a listed patent for which a certification has been submitted under subsection (b)(2)(A)(iv) or (j)(2)(A)(vii)(IV) of section 505, and in the patent infringement litigation resulting from the certification the court determines that the patent is valid and would be infringed, the period during which an application may not be approved under section 505(c)(3) or section 505(j)(4)(B) shall be extended by a period of six months after the date the patent expires (including any patent extensions).

"(d) CONDUCT OF PEDIATRIC STUDIES.—

"(1) AGREEMENT FOR STUDIES.—The Secretary may, pursuant to a written request from the Secretary under subsection (a) or (c), after consultation with—

"(A) the sponsor of an application for an investigational new drug under section 505(i);

"(B) the sponsor of an application for a new drug under section 505(b)(1); or

"(C) the holder of an approved application for a drug under section 505(b)(1),

agree with the sponsor or holder for the conduct of pediatric studies for such drug. Such agreement shall be in writing and shall include a timeframe for such studies.

"(2) WRITTEN PROTOCOLS TO MEET THE STUDIES REQUIREMENT.—If the sponsor or holder and the Secretary agree upon written protocols for the studies, the studies requirement of subsection (a) or (c) is satisfied upon the completion of the studies and submission of the reports thereof in accordance with the original written request and the written agreement referred to in paragraph (1). Not later than 60 days after the submission of the report of the studies, the Secretary shall determine if such studies were or were not conducted in accordance with the original written request and the written agreement and reported in accordance with the requirements of the Secretary for filing and so notify the sponsor or holder.

"(3) OTHER METHODS TO MEET THE STUDIES REQUIREMENT.—If the sponsor or holder and the Secretary have not agreed in writing on the protocols for the studies, the studies requirement of subsection (a) or (c) is satisfied when such studies have been completed and the reports accepted by the Secretary. Not later than 90 days after the submission of the reports of the studies, the Secretary shall accept or reject such reports and so notify the sponsor or holder. The Secretary's only responsibility in accepting or rejecting the reports shall be to determine, within the 90 days, whether the studies fairly respond to the written request, have been conducted in accordance with commonly accepted scientific principles and protocols, and have been reported in accordance with the requirements of the Secretary for filing.

"(e) DELAY OF EFFECTIVE DATE FOR CERTAIN APPLICATION.— If the Secretary determines that the acceptance or approval of an application under section 505(b)(2) or 505(j) for a new drug may occur after submission of reports of pediatric studies under this section, which were submitted prior to the expiration of the patent (including any patent extension) or the applicable period under clauses (ii) through (iv) of section 505(c)(3)(D) or clauses (ii) through (iv) of section 505(j)(4)(D), but before the Secretary has determined whether the requirements of subsection (d) have been satisfied, the Secretary shall delay the acceptance or approval under section 505(b)(2) or 505(j) until the determination under subsection (d) is made, but any such delay shall not exceed 90 days. In the event that requirements of this section are satisfied, the applicable six-month period under subsection (a) or (c) shall be deemed to have been running during the period of delay.

"(f) NOTICE OF DETERMINATIONS ON STUDIES REQUIREMENT.— The Secretary shall publish a notice of any determination that the requirements of subsection (d) have been met and that submissions and approvals under subsection (b)(2) or (j) of section 505 for a drug will be subject to the provisions of this section.

"(g) DEFINITIONS.—As used in this section, the term 'pediatric studies' or 'studies' means at least one clinical investigation (that, at the Secretary's discretion, may include pharmacokinetic studies) in pediatric age groups in which a drug is anticipated to be used.

"(h) LIMITATIONS.—A drug to which the six-month period under subsection (a) or (b) has already been applied—

"(1) may receive an additional six-month period under subsection (c)(1)(A)(ii) for a supplemental application if all other requirements under this section are satisfied, except that such a drug may not receive any additional such period under subsection (c)(2); and

"(2) may not receive any additional such period under subsection (c)(1)(B).

"(i) RELATIONSHIP TO REGULATIONS.—Notwithstanding any other provision of law, if any pediatric study is required pursuant to regulations promulgated by the Secretary and such study meets the completeness, timeliness, and other requirements of this section, such study shall be deemed to satisfy the requirement for market exclusivity pursuant to this section.

"(j) SUNSET.—A drug may not receive any six-month period under subsection (a) or (c) unless the application for the drug under section 505(b)(1) is submitted on or before January 1, 2002. After January 1, 2002, a drug shall receive a six-month period under subsection (c) if—

"(1) the drug was in commercial distribution as of the date of enactment of the Food and Drug Administration Modernization Act of 1997;

"(2) the drug was included by the Secretary on the list under subsection (b) as of January 1, 2002;

"(3) the Secretary determines that there is a continuing need for information relating to the use of the drug in the pediatric population and that the drug may provide health benefits in that population; and

"(4) all requirements of this section are met.

"(k) REPORT.—The Secretary shall conduct a study and report to Congress not later than January 1, 2001, based on the experience under the program established under this section. The study and report shall examine all relevant issues, including—

"(1) the effectiveness of the program in improving information about important pediatric uses for approved drugs;

"(2) the adequacy of the incentive provided under this section;

"(3) the economic impact of the program on taxpayers and consumers, including the impact of the lack of lower cost generic drugs on patients, including on lower income patients; and

"(4) any suggestions for modification that the Secretary determines to be appropriate.".

SEC. 112. EXPEDITING STUDY AND APPROVAL OF FAST TRACK DRUGS.

(a) IN GENERAL.—Chapter V (21 U.S.C. 351 et seq.), as amended by section 125, is amended by inserting before section 508 the following:

"SEC. 506. FAST TRACK PRODUCTS.

21 USC 356.

"(a) DESIGNATION OF DRUG AS A FAST TRACK PRODUCT.—

"(1) IN GENERAL.—The Secretary shall, at the request of the sponsor of a new drug, facilitate the development and expedite the review of such drug if it is intended for the treatment of a serious or life-threatening condition and it demonstrates the potential to address unmet medical needs for such a condition. (In this section, such a drug is referred to as a 'fast track product'.)

"(2) REQUEST FOR DESIGNATION.—The sponsor of a new drug may request the Secretary to designate the drug as a fast track product. A request for the designation may be made concurrently with, or at any time after, submission of an application for the investigation of the drug under section 505(i) or section 351(a)(3) of the Public Health Service Act.

"(3) DESIGNATION.—Within 60 calendar days after the receipt of a request under paragraph (2), the Secretary shall determine whether the drug that is the subject of the request meets the criteria described in paragraph (1). If the Secretary finds that the drug meets the criteria, the Secretary shall designate the drug as a fast track product and shall take such actions as are appropriate to expedite the development and review of the application for approval of such product.

"(b) APPROVAL OF APPLICATION FOR A FAST TRACK PRODUCT.—

"(1) IN GENERAL.—The Secretary may approve an application for approval of a fast track product under section 505(c) or section 351 of the Public Health Service Act upon a determination that the product has an effect on a clinical endpoint or on a surrogate endpoint that is reasonably likely to predict clinical benefit.

"(2) LIMITATION.—Approval of a fast track product under this subsection may be subject to the requirements—

"(A) that the sponsor conduct appropriate post-approval studies to validate the surrogate endpoint or otherwise confirm the effect on the clinical endpoint; and

"(B) that the sponsor submit copies of all promotional materials related to the fast track product during the preapproval review period and, following approval and for such period thereafter as the Secretary determines to be appropriate, at least 30 days prior to dissemination of the materials.

"(3) EXPEDITED WITHDRAWAL OF APPROVAL.—The Secretary may withdraw approval of a fast track product using expedited procedures (as prescribed by the Secretary in regulations which shall include an opportunity for an informal hearing) if—

"(A) the sponsor fails to conduct any required post-approval study of the fast track drug with due diligence;

"(B) a post-approval study of the fast track product fails to verify clinical benefit of the product;

"(C) other evidence demonstrates that the fast track product is not safe or effective under the conditions of use; or

"(D) the sponsor disseminates false or misleading promotional materials with respect to the product.

"(c) REVIEW OF INCOMPLETE APPLICATIONS FOR APPROVAL OF A FAST TRACK PRODUCT.—

"(1) IN GENERAL.—If the Secretary determines, after preliminary evaluation of clinical data submitted by the sponsor, that a fast track product may be effective, the Secretary shall evaluate for filing, and may commence review of portions of, an application for the approval of the product before the sponsor submits a complete application. The Secretary shall commence such review only if the applicant—

"(A) provides a schedule for submission of information necessary to make the application complete; and

"(B) pays any fee that may be required under section 736.

"(2) EXCEPTION.—Any time period for review of human drug applications that has been agreed to by the Secretary and that has been set forth in goals identified in letters of the Secretary (relating to the use of fees collected under section 736 to expedite the drug development process and the review of human drug applications) shall not apply to an application submitted under paragraph (1) until the date on which the application is complete.

"(d) AWARENESS EFFORTS.—The Secretary shall—

"(1) develop and disseminate to physicians, patient organizations, pharmaceutical and biotechnology companies, and other appropriate persons a description of the provisions of this section applicable to fast track products; and

"(2) establish a program to encourage the development of surrogate endpoints that are reasonably likely to predict clinical benefit for serious or life-threatening conditions for which there exist significant unmet medical needs.".

21 USC 356 note.   (b) GUIDANCE.—Within 1 year after the date of enactment of this Act, the Secretary of Health and Human Services shall issue guidance for fast track products (as defined in section 506(a)(1) of the Federal Food, Drug, and Cosmetic Act) that describes the policies and procedures that pertain to section 506 of such Act.

SEC. 113. INFORMATION PROGRAM ON CLINICAL TRIALS FOR SERIOUS OR LIFE-THREATENING DISEASES.

(a) IN GENERAL.—Section 402 of the Public Health Service Act (42 U.S.C. 282) is amended—

(1) by redesignating subsections (j) and (k) as subsections (k) and (l), respectively; and

(2) by inserting after subsection (i) the following:

"(j)(1)(A) The Secretary, acting through the Director of NIH, shall establish, maintain, and operate a data bank of information on clinical trials for drugs for serious or life-threatening diseases and conditions (in this subsection referred to as the 'data bank'). The activities of the data bank shall be integrated and coordinated with related activities of other agencies of the Department of Health and Human Services, and to the extent practicable, coordinated with other data banks containing similar information.

Establishment.

"(B) The Secretary shall establish the data bank after consultation with the Commissioner of Food and Drugs, the directors of the appropriate agencies of the National Institutes of Health (including the National Library of Medicine), and the Director of the Centers for Disease Control and Prevention.

"(2) In carrying out paragraph (1), the Secretary shall collect, catalog, store, and disseminate the information described in such paragraph. The Secretary shall disseminate such information through information systems, which shall include toll-free telephone communications, available to individuals with serious or life-threatening diseases and conditions, to other members of the public, to health care providers, and to researchers.

"(3) The data bank shall include the following:

"(A) A registry of clinical trials (whether federally or privately funded) of experimental treatments for serious or life-threatening diseases and conditions under regulations promulgated pursuant to section 505(i) of the Federal Food, Drug, and Cosmetic Act, which provides a description of the purpose of each experimental drug, either with the consent of the protocol sponsor, or when a trial to test effectiveness begins. Information provided shall consist of eligibility criteria for participation in the clinical trials, a description of the location of trial sites, and a point of contact for those wanting to enroll in the trial, and shall be in a form that can be readily understood by members of the public. Such information shall be forwarded to the data bank by the sponsor of the trial not later than 21 days after the approval of the protocol.

"(B) Information pertaining to experimental treatments for serious or life-threatening diseases and conditions that may be available—

"(i) under a treatment investigational new drug application that has been submitted to the Secretary under section 561(c) of the Federal Food, Drug, and Cosmetic Act; or

"(ii) as a Group C cancer drug (as defined by the National Cancer Institute).

The data bank may also include information pertaining to the results of clinical trials of such treatments, with the consent of the sponsor, including information concerning potential toxicities or adverse effects associated with the use or administration of such experimental treatments.

"(4) The data bank shall not include information relating to an investigation if the sponsor has provided a detailed certification to the Secretary that disclosure of such information would substantially interfere with the timely enrollment of subjects in the investigation, unless the Secretary, after the receipt of the certification, provides the sponsor with a detailed written determination that such disclosure would not substantially interfere with such enrollment.

Appropriation
authorization.

"(5) For the purpose of carrying out this subsection, there are authorized to be appropriated such sums as may be necessary. Fees collected under section 736 of the Federal Food, Drug, and Cosmetic Act shall not be used in carrying out this subsection.".

42 USC 282 note.

(b) COLLABORATION AND REPORT.—

(1) IN GENERAL.—The Secretary of Health and Human Services, the Director of the National Institutes of Health, and the Commissioner of Food and Drugs shall collaborate to determine the feasibility of including device investigations within the scope of the data bank under section 402(j) of the Public Health Service Act.

(2) REPORT.—Not later than two years after the date of enactment of this section, the Secretary of Health and Human Services shall prepare and submit to the Committee on Labor and Human Resources of the Senate and the Committee on Commerce of the House of Representatives a report—

(A) of the public health need, if any, for inclusion of device investigations within the scope of the data bank under section 402(j) of the Public Health Service Act;

(B) on the adverse impact, if any, on device innovation and research in the United States if information relating to such device investigations is required to be publicly disclosed; and

(C) on such other issues relating to such section 402(j) as the Secretary determines to be appropriate.

SEC. 114. HEALTH CARE ECONOMIC INFORMATION.

(a) IN GENERAL.—Section 502(a) (21 U.S.C. 352(a)) is amended by adding at the end the following: "Health care economic information provided to a formulary committee, or other similar entity, in the course of the committee or the entity carrying out its responsibilities for the selection of drugs for managed care or other similar organizations, shall not be considered to be false or misleading under this paragraph if the health care economic information directly relates to an indication approved under section 505 or under section 351(a) of the Public Health Service Act for such drug and is based on competent and reliable scientific evidence. The requirements set forth in section 505(a) or in section 351(a) of the Public Health Service Act shall not apply to health care economic information provided to such a committee or entity in accordance with this paragraph. Information that is relevant to the substantiation of the health care economic information presented pursuant to this paragraph shall be made available to the Secretary upon request. In this paragraph, the term 'health care economic information' means any analysis that identifies, measures, or compares the economic consequences, including the costs of the represented health outcomes, of the use of a drug to the use of another drug, to another health care intervention, or to no intervention.".

21 USC 352 note.

(b) STUDY AND REPORT.—The Comptroller General of the United States shall conduct a study of the implementation of the provisions added by the amendment made by subsection (a). Not later than 4 years and 6 months after the date of enactment of this Act, the Comptroller General of the United States shall prepare and submit to Congress a report containing the findings of the study.

SEC. 115. CLINICAL INVESTIGATIONS.

(a) CLARIFICATION OF THE NUMBER OF REQUIRED CLINICAL INVESTIGATIONS FOR APPROVAL.—Section 505(d) (21 U.S.C. 355(d)) is amended by adding at the end the following: "If the Secretary determines, based on relevant science, that data from one adequate and well-controlled clinical investigation and confirmatory evidence (obtained prior to or after such investigation) are sufficient to establish effectiveness, the Secretary may consider such data and evidence to constitute substantial evidence for purposes of the preceding sentence.".

(b) WOMEN AND MINORITIES.—Section 505(b)(1) (21 U.S.C. 355(b)(1)) is amended by adding at the end the following: "The Secretary shall, in consultation with the Director of the National Institutes of Health and with representatives of the drug manufacturing industry, review and develop guidance, as appropriate, on the inclusion of women and minorities in clinical trials required by clause (A).".

SEC. 116. MANUFACTURING CHANGES FOR DRUGS.

(a) IN GENERAL.—Chapter V, as amended by section 112, is amended by inserting after section 506 the following section:

"SEC. 506A. MANUFACTURING CHANGES.   21 USC 356a.

"(a) IN GENERAL.—With respect to a drug for which there is in effect an approved application under section 505 or 512 or a license under section 351 of the Public Health Service Act, a change from the manufacturing process approved pursuant to such application or license may be made, and the drug as made with the change may be distributed, if—

"(1) the holder of the approved application or license (referred to in this section as a 'holder') has validated the effects of the change in accordance with subsection (b); and

"(2)(A) in the case of a major manufacturing change, the holder has complied with the requirements of subsection (c); or

"(B) in the case of a change that is not a major manufacturing change, the holder complies with the applicable requirements of subsection (d).

"(b) VALIDATION OF EFFECTS OF CHANGES.—For purposes of subsection (a)(1), a drug made with a manufacturing change (whether a major manufacturing change or otherwise) may be distributed only if, before distribution of the drug as so made, the holder involved validates the effects of the change on the identity, strength, quality, purity, and potency of the drug as the identity, strength, quality, purity, and potency may relate to the safety or effectiveness of the drug.

"(c) MAJOR MANUFACTURING CHANGES.—

"(1) REQUIREMENT OF SUPPLEMENTAL APPLICATION.—For purposes of subsection (a)(2)(A), a drug made with a major manufacturing change may be distributed only if, before the distribution of the drug as so made, the holder involved submits to the Secretary a supplemental application for such change and the Secretary approves the application. The application shall contain such information as the Secretary determines to be appropriate, and shall include the information developed under subsection (b) by the holder in validating the effects of the change.

"(2) CHANGES QUALIFYING AS MAJOR CHANGES.—For purposes of subsection (a)(2)(A), a major manufacturing change is a manufacturing change that is determined by the Secretary to have substantial potential to adversely affect the identity, strength, quality, purity, or potency of the drug as they may relate to the safety or effectiveness of a drug. Such a change includes a change that—

"(A) is made in the qualitative or quantitative formulation of the drug involved or in the specifications in the approved application or license referred to in subsection (a) for the drug (unless exempted by the Secretary by regulation or guidance from the requirements of this subsection);

"(B) is determined by the Secretary by regulation or guidance to require completion of an appropriate clinical study demonstrating equivalence of the drug to the drug as manufactured without the change; or

"(C) is another type of change determined by the Secretary by regulation or guidance to have a substantial potential to adversely affect the safety or effectiveness of the drug.

"(d) OTHER MANUFACTURING CHANGES.—

"(1) IN GENERAL.—For purposes of subsection (a)(2)(B), the Secretary may regulate drugs made with manufacturing changes that are not major manufacturing changes as follows:

"(A) The Secretary may in accordance with paragraph (2) authorize holders to distribute such drugs without submitting a supplemental application for such changes.

"(B) The Secretary may in accordance with paragraph (3) require that, prior to the distribution of such drugs, holders submit to the Secretary supplemental applications for such changes.

"(C) The Secretary may establish categories of such changes and designate categories to which subparagraph (A) applies and categories to which subparagraph (B) applies.

"(2) CHANGES NOT REQUIRING SUPPLEMENTAL APPLICATION.—

"(A) SUBMISSION OF REPORT.—A holder making a manufacturing change to which paragraph (1)(A) applies shall submit to the Secretary a report on the change, which shall contain such information as the Secretary determines to be appropriate, and which shall include the information developed under subsection (b) by the holder in validating the effects of the change. The report shall be submitted by such date as the Secretary may specify.

"(B) AUTHORITY REGARDING ANNUAL REPORTS.—In the case of a holder that during a single year makes more than one manufacturing change to which paragraph (1)(A) applies, the Secretary may in carrying out subparagraph (A) authorize the holder to comply with such subparagraph by submitting a single report for the year that provides the information required in such subparagraph for all the changes made by the holder during the year.

"(3) CHANGES REQUIRING SUPPLEMENTAL APPLICATION.—

"(A) SUBMISSION OF SUPPLEMENTAL APPLICATION.—The supplemental application required under paragraph (1)(B) for a manufacturing change shall contain such information as the Secretary determines to be appropriate, which shall include the information developed under subsection (b) by the holder in validating the effects of the change.

"(B) AUTHORITY FOR DISTRIBUTION.—In the case of a manufacturing change to which paragraph (1)(B) applies:

"(i) The holder involved may commence distribution of the drug involved 30 days after the Secretary receives the supplemental application under such paragraph, unless the Secretary notifies the holder within such 30-day period that prior approval of the application is required before distribution may be commenced.

"(ii) The Secretary may designate a category of such changes for the purpose of providing that, in the case of a change that is in such category, the holder involved may commence distribution of the drug involved upon the receipt by the Secretary of a supplemental application for the change.

"(iii) If the Secretary disapproves the supplemental application, the Secretary may order the manufacturer to cease the distribution of the drugs that have been made with the manufacturing change.".

(b) TRANSITION RULE.—The amendment made by subsection (a) takes effect upon the effective date of regulations promulgated by the Secretary of Health and Human Services to implement such amendment, or upon the expiration of the 24-month period beginning on the date of the enactment of this Act, whichever occurs first.

21 USC 356a note.

SEC. 117. STREAMLINING CLINICAL RESEARCH ON DRUGS.

Section 505(i) (21 U.S.C. 355(i)) is amended—

(1) by redesignating paragraphs (1) through (3) as subparagraphs (A) through (C), respectively;

(2) by inserting "(1)" after "(i)";

(3) by striking the last two sentences; and

(4) by inserting after paragraph (1) (as designated by paragraph (2) of this section) the following new paragraphs:

"(2) Subject to paragraph (3), a clinical investigation of a new drug may begin 30 days after the Secretary has received from the manufacturer or sponsor of the investigation a submission containing such information about the drug and the clinical investigation, including—

"(A) information on design of the investigation and adequate reports of basic information, certified by the applicant to be accurate reports, necessary to assess the safety of the drug for use in clinical investigation; and

"(B) adequate information on the chemistry and manufacturing of the drug, controls available for the drug, and primary data tabulations from animal or human studies.

"(3)(A) At any time, the Secretary may prohibit the sponsor of an investigation from conducting the investigation (referred to in this paragraph as a 'clinical hold') if the Secretary makes a determination described in subparagraph (B). The Secretary shall specify the basis for the clinical hold, including the specific information available to the Secretary which served as the basis for such clinical hold, and confirm such determination in writing.

"(B) For purposes of subparagraph (A), a determination described in this subparagraph with respect to a clinical hold is that—

"(i) the drug involved represents an unreasonable risk to the safety of the persons who are the subjects of the clinical investigation, taking into account the qualifications of the clinical investigators, information about the drug, the design of the clinical investigation, the condition for which the drug is to be investigated, and the health status of the subjects involved; or

"(ii) the clinical hold should be issued for such other reasons as the Secretary may by regulation establish (including reasons established by regulation before the date of the enactment of the Food and Drug Administration Modernization Act of 1997).

"(C) Any written request to the Secretary from the sponsor of an investigation that a clinical hold be removed shall receive a decision, in writing and specifying the reasons therefor, within 30 days after receipt of such request. Any such request shall include sufficient information to support the removal of such clinical hold.

"(4) Regulations under paragraph (1) shall provide that such exemption shall be conditioned upon the manufacturer, or the sponsor of the investigation, requiring that experts using such drugs for investigational purposes certify to such manufacturer or sponsor that they will inform any human beings to whom such drugs, or any controls used in connection therewith, are being administered, or their representatives, that such drugs are being used for investigational purposes and will obtain the consent of such human beings or their representatives, except where it is not feasible or it is contrary to the best interests of such human beings. Nothing in this subsection shall be construed to require any clinical investigator to submit directly to the Secretary reports on the investigational use of drugs.".

21 USC 355 note.

SEC. 118. DATA REQUIREMENTS FOR DRUGS AND BIOLOGICS.

Within 12 months after the date of enactment of this Act, the Secretary of Health and Human Services, acting through the Commissioner of Food and Drugs, shall issue guidance that describes when abbreviated study reports may be submitted, in lieu of full reports, with a new drug application under section 505(b) of the Federal Food, Drug, and Cosmetic Act (21 U.S.C. 355(b)) and with a biologics license application under section 351 of the Public Health Service Act (42 U.S.C. 262) for certain types of studies. Such guidance shall describe the kinds of studies for which abbreviated reports are appropriate and the appropriate abbreviated report formats.

SEC. 119. CONTENT AND REVIEW OF APPLICATIONS.

(a) SECTION 505(b).—Section 505(b) (21 U.S.C. 355(b)) is amended by adding at the end the following:

"(4)(A) The Secretary shall issue guidance for the individuals who review applications submitted under paragraph (1) or under section 351 of the Public Health Service Act, which shall relate to promptness in conducting the review, technical excellence, lack of bias and conflict of interest, and knowledge of regulatory and scientific standards, and which shall apply equally to all individuals who review such applications.

"(B) The Secretary shall meet with a sponsor of an investigation or an applicant for approval for a drug under this subsection or section 351 of the Public Health Service Act if the sponsor or applicant makes a reasonable written request for a meeting for the purpose of reaching agreement on the design and size of clinical trials intended to form the primary basis of an effectiveness claim. The sponsor or applicant shall provide information necessary for discussion and agreement on the design and size of the clinical trials. Minutes of any such meeting shall be prepared by the Secretary and made available to the sponsor or applicant upon request.

"(C) Any agreement regarding the parameters of the design and size of clinical trials of a new drug under this paragraph that is reached between the Secretary and a sponsor or applicant shall be reduced to writing and made part of the administrative record by the Secretary. Such agreement shall not be changed after the testing begins, except—

"(i) with the written agreement of the sponsor or applicant; or

"(ii) pursuant to a decision, made in accordance with subparagraph (D) by the director of the reviewing division, that a substantial scientific issue essential to determining the safety or effectiveness of the drug has been identified after the testing has begun.

"(D) A decision under subparagraph (C)(ii) by the director shall be in writing and the Secretary shall provide to the sponsor or applicant an opportunity for a meeting at which the director and the sponsor or applicant will be present and at which the director will document the scientific issue involved.

"(E) The written decisions of the reviewing division shall be binding upon, and may not directly or indirectly be changed by, the field or compliance division personnel unless such field or compliance division personnel demonstrate to the reviewing division why such decision should be modified.

"(F) No action by the reviewing division may be delayed because of the unavailability of information from or action by field personnel unless the reviewing division determines that a delay is necessary to assure the marketing of a safe and effective drug.

"(G) For purposes of this paragraph, the reviewing division is the division responsible for the review of an application for approval of a drug under this subsection or section 351 of the Public Health Service Act (including all scientific and medical matters, chemistry, manufacturing, and controls).".

(b) SECTION 505(j).—

(1) AMENDMENT.—Section 505(j) (21 U.S.C 355(j)) is amended—

(A) by redesignating paragraphs (3) through (8) as paragraphs (4) through (9), respectively; and

(B) by adding after paragraph (2) the following:

"(3)(A) The Secretary shall issue guidance for the individuals who review applications submitted under paragraph (1), which shall relate to promptness in conducting the review, technical excellence, lack of bias and conflict of interest, and knowledge of regulatory and scientific standards, and which shall apply equally to all individuals who review such applications.

"(B) The Secretary shall meet with a sponsor of an investigation or an applicant for approval for a drug under this subsection if the sponsor or applicant makes a reasonable written request for a meeting for the purpose of reaching agreement on the design and size of bioavailability and bioequivalence studies needed for approval of such application. The sponsor or applicant shall provide information necessary for discussion and agreement on the design and size of such studies. Minutes of any such meeting shall be prepared by the Secretary and made available to the sponsor or applicant.

"(C) Any agreement regarding the parameters of design and size of bioavailability and bioequivalence studies of a drug under this paragraph that is reached between the Secretary and a sponsor or applicant shall be reduced to writing and made part of the administrative record by the Secretary. Such agreement shall not be changed after the testing begins, except—

"(i) with the written agreement of the sponsor or applicant; or

"(ii) pursuant to a decision, made in accordance with subparagraph (D) by the director of the reviewing division, that a substantial scientific issue essential to determining the safety or effectiveness of the drug has been identified after the testing has begun.

"(D) A decision under subparagraph (C)(ii) by the director shall be in writing and the Secretary shall provide to the sponsor or applicant an opportunity for a meeting at which the director and the sponsor or applicant will be present and at which the director will document the scientific issue involved.

"(E) The written decisions of the reviewing division shall be binding upon, and may not directly or indirectly be changed by, the field or compliance office personnel unless such field or compliance office personnel demonstrate to the reviewing division why such decision should be modified.

"(F) No action by the reviewing division may be delayed because of the unavailability of information from or action by field personnel unless the reviewing division determines that a delay is necessary to assure the marketing of a safe and effective drug.

"(G) For purposes of this paragraph, the reviewing division is the division responsible for the review of an application for approval of a drug under this subsection (including scientific matters, chemistry, manufacturing, and controls).".

(2) CONFORMING AMENDMENTS.—Section 505(j) (21 U.S.C. 355(j)), as amended by paragraph (1), is further amended—

(A) in paragraph (2)(A)(i), by striking "(6)" and inserting "(7)";

(B) in paragraph (4) (as redesignated in paragraph (1)), by striking "(4)" and inserting "(5)";

(C) in paragraph (4)(I) (as redesignated in paragraph (1)), by striking "(5)" and inserting "(6)"; and

(D) in paragraph (7)(C) (as redesignated in paragraph (1)), by striking "(5)" each place it occurs and inserting "(6)".

SEC. 120. SCIENTIFIC ADVISORY PANELS.

Section 505 (21 U.S.C. 355) is amended by adding at the end the following:

"(n)(1) For the purpose of providing expert scientific advice and recommendations to the Secretary regarding a clinical investigation of a drug or the approval for marketing of a drug under section 505 or section 351 of the Public Health Service Act, the

Secretary shall establish panels of experts or use panels of experts established before the date of enactment of the Food and Drug Administration Modernization Act of 1997, or both.

"(2) The Secretary may delegate the appointment and oversight authority granted under section 904 to a director of a center or successor entity within the Food and Drug Administration.

"(3) The Secretary shall make appointments to each panel established under paragraph (1) so that each panel shall consist of—

"(A) members who are qualified by training and experience to evaluate the safety and effectiveness of the drugs to be referred to the panel and who, to the extent feasible, possess skill and experience in the development, manufacture, or utilization of such drugs;

"(B) members with diverse expertise in such fields as clinical and administrative medicine, pharmacy, pharmacology, pharmacoeconomics, biological and physical sciences, and other related professions;

"(C) a representative of consumer interests, and a representative of interests of the drug manufacturing industry not directly affected by the matter to be brought before the panel; and

"(D) two or more members who are specialists or have other expertise in the particular disease or condition for which the drug under review is proposed to be indicated.

Scientific, trade, and consumer organizations shall be afforded an opportunity to nominate individuals for appointment to the panels. No individual who is in the regular full-time employ of the United States and engaged in the administration of this Act may be a voting member of any panel. The Secretary shall designate one of the members of each panel to serve as chairman thereof.

"(4) Each member of a panel shall publicly disclose all conflicts of interest that member may have with the work to be undertaken by the panel. No member of a panel may vote on any matter where the member or the immediate family of such member could gain financially from the advice given to the Secretary. The Secretary may grant a waiver of any conflict of interest requirement upon public disclosure of such conflict of interest if such waiver is necessary to afford the panel essential expertise, except that the Secretary may not grant a waiver for a member of a panel when the member's own scientific work is involved.

"(5) The Secretary shall, as appropriate, provide education and training to each new panel member before such member participates in a panel's activities, including education regarding requirements under this Act and related regulations of the Secretary, and the administrative processes and procedures related to panel meetings.

"(6) Panel members (other than officers or employees of the United States), while attending meetings or conferences of a panel or otherwise engaged in its business, shall be entitled to receive compensation for each day so engaged, including traveltime, at rates to be fixed by the Secretary, but not to exceed the daily equivalent of the rate in effect for positions classified above grade GS–15 of the General Schedule. While serving away from their homes or regular places of business, panel members may be allowed travel expenses (including per diem in lieu of subsistence) as authorized by section 5703 of title 5, United States Code, for persons in the Government service employed intermittently.

"(7) The Secretary shall ensure that scientific advisory panels meet regularly and at appropriate intervals so that any matter to be reviewed by such a panel can be presented to the panel not more than 60 days after the matter is ready for such review. Meetings of the panel may be held using electronic communication to convene the meetings.

"(8) Within 90 days after a scientific advisory panel makes recommendations on any matter under its review, the Food and Drug Administration official responsible for the matter shall review the conclusions and recommendations of the panel, and notify the affected persons of the final decision on the matter, or of the reasons that no such decision has been reached. Each such final decision shall be documented including the rationale for the decision.".

SEC. 121. POSITRON EMISSION TOMOGRAPHY.

(a) REGULATION OF COMPOUNDED POSITRON EMISSION TOMOGRAPHY DRUGS.—Section 201 (21 U.S.C. 321) is amended by adding at the end the following:

"(ii) The term 'compounded positron emission tomography drug'—

"(1) means a drug that—

"(A) exhibits spontaneous disintegration of unstable nuclei by the emission of positrons and is used for the purpose of providing dual photon positron emission tomographic diagnostic images; and

"(B) has been compounded by or on the order of a practitioner who is licensed by a State to compound or order compounding for a drug described in subparagraph (A), and is compounded in accordance with that State's law, for a patient or for research, teaching, or quality control; and

"(2) includes any nonradioactive reagent, reagent kit, ingredient, nuclide generator, accelerator, target material, electronic synthesizer, or other apparatus or computer program to be used in the preparation of such a drug.".

(b) ADULTERATION.—

(1) IN GENERAL.—Section 501(a) (21 U.S.C. 351(a)) is amended by striking "; or (3)" and inserting the following: "; or (C) if it is a compounded positron emission tomography drug and the methods used in, or the facilities and controls used for, its compounding, processing, packing, or holding do not conform to or are not operated or administered in conformity with the positron emission tomography compounding standards and the official monographs of the United States Pharmacopoeia to assure that such drug meets the requirements of this Act as to safety and has the identity and strength, and meets the quality and purity characteristics, that it purports or is represented to possess; or (3)".

21 USC 351 note.

(2) SUNSET.—Section 501(a)(2)(C) of the Federal Food, Drug, and Cosmetic Act (21 U.S.C. 351(a)(2)(C)) shall not apply 4 years after the date of enactment of this Act or 2 years after the date on which the Secretary of Health and Human Services establishes the requirements described in subsection (c)(1)(B), whichever is later.

(c) REQUIREMENTS FOR REVIEW OF APPROVAL PROCEDURES AND CURRENT GOOD MANUFACTURING PRACTICES FOR POSITRON EMISSION TOMOGRAPHY.—

21 USC 355 note.

(1) PROCEDURES AND REQUIREMENTS.—

(A) IN GENERAL.—In order to take account of the special characteristics of positron emission tomography drugs and the special techniques and processes required to produce these drugs, not later than 2 years after the date of enactment of this Act, the Secretary of Health and Human Services shall establish—

(i) appropriate procedures for the approval of positron emission tomography drugs pursuant to section 505 of the Federal Food, Drug, and Cosmetic Act (21 U.S.C. 355); and

(ii) appropriate current good manufacturing practice requirements for such drugs.

(B) CONSIDERATIONS AND CONSULTATION.—In establishing the procedures and requirements required by subparagraph (A), the Secretary of Health and Human Services shall take due account of any relevant differences between not-for-profit institutions that compound the drugs for their patients and commercial manufacturers of the drugs. Prior to establishing the procedures and requirements, the Secretary of Health and Human Services shall consult with patient advocacy groups, professional associations, manufacturers, and physicians and scientists licensed to make or use positron emission tomography drugs.

(2) SUBMISSION OF NEW DRUG APPLICATIONS AND ABBREVIATED NEW DRUG APPLICATIONS.—

(A) IN GENERAL.—Except as provided in subparagraph (B), the Secretary of Health and Human Services shall not require the submission of new drug applications or abbreviated new drug applications under subsection (b) or (j) of section 505 (21 U.S.C. 355), for compounded positron emission tomography drugs that are not adulterated drugs described in section 501(a)(2)(C) of the Federal Food, Drug, and Cosmetic Act (21 U.S.C. 351(a)(2)(C)) (as amended by subsection (b)), for a period of 4 years after the date of enactment of this Act, or for 2 years after the date on which the Secretary establishes procedures and requirements under paragraph (1), whichever is longer.

(B) EXCEPTION.—Nothing in this Act shall prohibit the voluntary submission of such applications or the review of such applications by the Secretary of Health and Human Services. Nothing in this Act shall constitute an exemption for a positron emission tomography drug from the requirements of regulations issued under section 505(i) of the Federal Food, Drug, and Cosmetic Act (21 U.S.C. 355(i)).

(d) REVOCATION OF CERTAIN INCONSISTENT DOCUMENTS.— Within 30 days after the date of enactment of this Act, the Secretary of Health and Human Services shall publish in the Federal Register a notice terminating the application of the following notices and rule:

Federal Register, publication.

(1) A notice entitled "Regulation of Positron Emission Tomography Radiopharmaceutical Drug Products; Guidance; Public Workshop", published in the Federal Register on February 27, 1995, 60 Fed. Reg. 10594.

(2) A notice entitled "Draft Guideline on the Manufacture of Positron Emission Tomography Radiopharmaceutical Drug Products; Availability", published in the Federal Register on February 27, 1995, 60 Fed. Reg. 10593.

(3) A final rule entitled "Current Good Manufacturing Practice for Finished Pharmaceuticals; Positron Emission Tomography", published in the Federal Register on April 22, 1997, 62 Fed. Reg. 19493 (codified at part 211 of title 21, Code of Federal Regulations).

21 USC 355 note.

(e) DEFINITION.—As used in this section, the term "compounded positron emission tomography drug" has the meaning given the term in section 201 of the Federal Food, Drug, and Cosmetic Act (21 U.S.C. 321).

21 USC 355 note.

SEC. 122. REQUIREMENTS FOR RADIOPHARMACEUTICALS.

(a) REQUIREMENTS.—
(1) REGULATIONS.—
(A) PROPOSED REGULATIONS.—Not later than 180 days after the date of enactment of this Act, the Secretary of Health and Human Services, after consultation with patient advocacy groups, associations, physicians licensed to use radiopharmaceuticals, and the regulated industry, shall issue proposed regulations governing the approval of radiopharmaceuticals. The regulations shall provide that the determination of the safety and effectiveness of such a radiopharmaceutical under section 505 of the Federal Food, Drug, and Cosmetic Act (21 U.S.C. 355) or section 351 of the Public Health Service Act (42 U.S.C. 262) shall include consideration of the proposed use of the radiopharmaceutical in the practice of medicine, the pharmacological and toxicological activity of the radiopharmaceutical (including any carrier or ligand component of the radiopharmaceutical), and the estimated absorbed radiation dose of the radiopharmaceutical.
(B) FINAL REGULATIONS.—Not later than 18 months after the date of enactment of this Act, the Secretary shall promulgate final regulations governing the approval of the radiopharmaceuticals.
(2) SPECIAL RULE.—In the case of a radiopharmaceutical, the indications for which such radiopharmaceutical is approved for marketing may, in appropriate cases, refer to manifestations of disease (such as biochemical, physiological, anatomic, or pathological processes) common to, or present in, one or more disease states.
(b) DEFINITION.—In this section, the term "radiopharmaceutical" means—
(1) an article—
(A) that is intended for use in the diagnosis or monitoring of a disease or a manifestation of a disease in humans; and
(B) that exhibits spontaneous disintegration of unstable nuclei with the emission of nuclear particles or photons; or
(2) any nonradioactive reagent kit or nuclide generator that is intended to be used in the preparation of any such article.

SEC. 123. MODERNIZATION OF REGULATION.

(a) LICENSES.—

(1) IN GENERAL.—Section 351(a) of the Public Health Service Act (42 U.S.C. 262(a)) is amended to read as follows:

"(a)(1) No person shall introduce or deliver for introduction into interstate commerce any biological product unless—

"(A) a biologics license is in effect for the biological product; and

"(B) each package of the biological product is plainly marked with—

"(i) the proper name of the biological product contained in the package;

"(ii) the name, address, and applicable license number of the manufacturer of the biological product; and

"(iii) the expiration date of the biological product.

"(2)(A) The Secretary shall establish, by regulation, requirements for the approval, suspension, and revocation of biologics licenses.

"(B) The Secretary shall approve a biologics license application—

"(i) on the basis of a demonstration that—

"(I) the biological product that is the subject of the application is safe, pure, and potent; and

"(II) the facility in which the biological product is manufactured, processed, packed, or held meets standards designed to assure that the biological product continues to be safe, pure, and potent; and

"(ii) if the applicant (or other appropriate person) consents to the inspection of the facility that is the subject of the application, in accordance with subsection (c).

"(3) The Secretary shall prescribe requirements under which a biological product undergoing investigation shall be exempt from the requirements of paragraph (1).".

(2) ELIMINATION OF EXISTING LICENSE REQUIREMENT.—Section 351(d) of the Public Health Service Act (42 U.S.C. 262(d)) is amended—

(A) by striking "(d)(1)" and all that follows through "of this section.";

(B) in paragraph (2)—

(i) by striking "(2)(A) Upon" and inserting "(d)(1) Upon" and

(ii) by redesignating subparagraph (B) as paragraph (2); and

(C) in paragraph (2) (as so redesignated by subparagraph (B)(ii))—

(i) by striking "subparagraph (A)" and inserting "paragraph (1)"; and

(ii) by striking "this subparagraph" each place it appears and inserting "this paragraph".

(b) LABELING.—Section 351(b) of the Public Health Service Act (42 U.S.C. 262(b)) is amended to read as follows:

"(b) No person shall falsely label or mark any package or container of any biological product or alter any label or mark on the package or container of the biological product so as to falsify the label or mark.".

(c) INSPECTION.—Section 351(c) of the Public Health Service Act (42 U.S.C. 262(c)) is amended by striking "virus, serum," and all that follows and inserting "biological product.".

(d) DEFINITION; APPLICATION.—Section 351 of the Public Health Service Act (42 U.S.C. 262) is amended by adding at the end the following:

"(i) In this section, the term 'biological product' means a virus, therapeutic serum, toxin, antitoxin, vaccine, blood, blood component or derivative, allergenic product, or analogous product, or arsphenamine or derivative of arsphenamine (or any other trivalent organic arsenic compound), applicable to the prevention, treatment, or cure of a disease or condition of human beings.".

(e) CONFORMING AMENDMENT.—Section 503(g)(4) (21 U.S.C. 353(g)(4)) is amended—

(1) in subparagraph (A)—

(A) by striking "section 351(a)" and inserting "section 351(i)"; and

(B) by striking "262(a)" and inserting "262(i)"; and

(2) in subparagraph (B)(iii), by striking "product or establishment license under subsection (a) or (d)" and inserting "biologics license application under subsection (a)".

21 USC 355 note.

(f) SPECIAL RULE.—The Secretary of Health and Human Services shall take measures to minimize differences in the review and approval of products required to have approved biologics license applications under section 351 of the Public Health Service Act (42 U.S.C. 262) and products required to have approved new drug applications under section 505(b)(1) of the Federal Food, Drug, and Cosmetic Act (21 U.S.C. 355(b)(1)).

(g) APPLICATION OF FEDERAL FOOD, DRUG, AND COSMETIC ACT.—Section 351 of the Public Health Service Act (42 U.S.C. 262), as amended by subsection (d), is further amended by adding at the end the following:

"(j) The Federal Food, Drug, and Cosmetic Act applies to a biological product subject to regulation under this section, except that a product for which a license has been approved under subsection (a) shall not be required to have an approved application under section 505 of such Act.".

(h) EXAMINATIONS AND PROCEDURES.—Paragraph (3) of section 353(d) of the Public Health Service Act (42 U.S.C. 263a(d)) is amended to read as follows:

"(3) EXAMINATIONS AND PROCEDURES.—The examinations and procedures identified in paragraph (2) are laboratory examinations and procedures that have been approved by the Food and Drug Administration for home use or that, as determined by the Secretary, are simple laboratory examinations and procedures that have an insignificant risk of an erroneous result, including those that—

"(A) employ methodologies that are so simple and accurate as to render the likelihood of erroneous results by the user negligible, or

"(B) the Secretary has determined pose no unreasonable risk of harm to the patient if performed incorrectly.".

SEC. 124. PILOT AND SMALL SCALE MANUFACTURE.

(a) HUMAN DRUGS.—Section 505(c) (21 U.S.C. 355(c)) is amended by adding at the end the following:

"(4) A drug manufactured in a pilot or other small facility may be used to demonstrate the safety and effectiveness of the drug and to obtain approval for the drug prior to manufacture of the drug in a larger facility, unless the Secretary makes a determination that a full scale production facility is necessary to ensure the safety or effectiveness of the drug.".

(b) ANIMAL DRUGS.—Section 512(c) (21 U.S.C. 360b(c)) is amended by adding at the end the following:

"(4) A drug manufactured in a pilot or other small facility may be used to demonstrate the safety and effectiveness of the drug and to obtain approval for the drug prior to manufacture of the drug in a larger facility, unless the Secretary makes a determination that a full scale production facility is necessary to ensure the safety or effectiveness of the drug.".

SEC. 125. INSULIN AND ANTIBIOTICS.

(a) CERTIFICATION OF DRUGS CONTAINING INSULIN.—

(1) AMENDMENT.—Section 506 (21 U.S.C. 356), as in effect before the date of the enactment of this Act, is repealed.

(2) CONFORMING AMENDMENTS.—

(A) Section 301(j) (21 U.S.C. 331(j)) is amended by striking "506, 507,".

(B) Subsection (k) of section 502 (21 U.S.C. 352) is repealed.

(C) Sections 301(i)(1), 510(j)(1)(A), and 510(j)(1)(D) (21 U.S.C. 331(i)(1), 360(j)(1)(A), 360(j)(1)(D)) are each amended by striking ", 506, 507,".

(D) Section 801(d)(1) (21 U.S.C. 381(d)(1)) is amended by inserting after "503(b)" the following: "or composed wholly or partly of insulin".

(E) Section 8126(h)(2) of title 38, United States Code, is amended by inserting "or" at the end of subparagraph (B), by striking "; or" at the end of subparagraph (C) and inserting a period, and by striking subparagraph (D).

(b) CERTIFICATION OF ANTIBIOTICS.—

(1) AMENDMENT.—Section 507 (21 U.S.C. 357) is repealed.

(2) CONFORMING AMENDMENTS.—

(A) Section 201(aa) (21 U.S.C. 321(aa)) is amended by striking out "or 507", section 201(dd) (21 U.S.C. 321(dd)) is amended by striking "507,", and section 201(ff)(3)(A) (21 U.S.C. 321(ff)(3)(A)) is amended by striking ", certified as an antibiotic under section 507,".

(B) Section 301(e) (21 U.S.C. 331(e)) is amended by striking "507(d) or (g),".

(C) Section 306(d)(4)(B)(ii) (21 U.S.C. 335a(d)(4)(B)(ii)) is amended by striking "or 507".

(D) Section 502 (21 U.S.C. 352) is amended by striking subsection (l).

(E) Section 520(l) (21 U.S.C. 360j(l)) is amended by striking paragraph (4) and by striking "or Antibiotic Drugs" in the subsection heading.

(F) Section 525(a) (21 U.S.C. 360aa(a)) is amended by inserting "or" at the end of paragraph (1), by striking paragraph (2), and by redesignating paragraph (3) as paragraph (2).

(G) Section 525(a) (21 U.S.C. 360aa(a)) is amended by striking ", certification of such drug for such disease or condition under section 507,".

(H) Section 526(a)(1) (21 U.S.C. 360bb) is amended by striking "the submission of an application for certification of the drug under section 507,", by inserting "or" at the end of subparagraph (A), by striking subparagraph (B), and by redesignating subparagraph (C) as subparagraph (B).

(I) Section 526(b) (21 U.S.C. 360bb(b)) is amended—

(i) in paragraph (1), by striking ", a certificate was issued for the drug under section 507,"; and

(ii) in paragraph (2) by striking ", a certificate has not been issued for the drug under section 507," and by striking ", approval of an application for certification under section 507,".

(J) Section 527(a) (21 U.S.C. 360cc(a)) is amended by inserting "or" at the end of paragraph (1), by striking paragraph (2), by redesignating paragraph (3) as paragraph (2), and by striking ", issue another certification under section 507,".

(K) Section 527(b) (21 U.S.C. 360cc(b)) is amended by striking ", if a certification is issued under section 507 for such a drug,", ", of the issuance of the certification under section 507,", ", issue another certification under section 507,", ", of such certification,", ", of the certification,", and ", issuance of other certifications,".

(L) Section 704(a)(1) (21 U.S.C. 374(a)(1)) is amended by striking ", section 507 (d) or (g),".

(M) Section 735(1) (21 U.S.C. 379g(1)(C)) is amended by inserting "or" at the end of subparagraph (B), by striking subparagraph (C), and by redesignating subparagraph (D) as subparagraph (C).

(N) Subparagraphs (A)(ii) and (B) of sections 5(b)(1) of the Orphan Drug Act (21 U.S.C. 360ee(b)(1)(A), 360ee(b)(1)(B)) are each amended by striking "or 507".

26 USC 45C.

(O) Section 45C(b)(2)(A)(ii)(II) of the Internal Revenue Code of 1986 is amended by striking "or 507".

(P) Section 156(f)(4)(B) of title 35, United States Code, is amended by striking "507," each place it occurs.

(c) EXPORTATION.—Section 802 (21 U.S.C. 382) is amended by adding at the end the following:

"(i) Insulin and antibiotic drugs may be exported without regard to the requirements in this section if the insulin and antibiotic drugs meet the requirements of section 801(e)(1).".

21 USC 355 note.

(d) TRANSITION.—

(1) IN GENERAL.—An application that was approved by the Secretary of Health and Human Services before the date of the enactment of this Act for the marketing of an antibiotic drug under section 507 of the Federal Food, Drug, and Cosmetic Act (21 U.S.C. 357), as in effect on the day before the date of the enactment of this Act, shall, on and after such date of enactment, be considered to be an application that was submitted and filed under section 505(b) of such Act (21 U.S.C. 355(b)) and approved for safety and effectiveness under section

505(c) of such Act (21 U.S.C. 355(c)), except that if such application for marketing was in the form of an abbreviated application, the application shall be considered to have been filed and approved under section 505(j) of such Act (21 U.S.C. 355(j)).

(2) EXCEPTION.—The following subsections of section 505 (21 U.S.C. 355) shall not apply to any application for marketing in which the drug that is the subject of the application contains an antibiotic drug and the antibiotic drug was the subject of any application for marketing received by the Secretary of Health and Human Services under section 507 of such Act (21 U.S.C. 357) before the date of the enactment of this Act:

(A)(i) Subsections (c)(2), (d)(6), (e)(4), (j)(2)(A)(vii), (j)(2)(A)(viii), (j)(2)(B), (j)(4)(B), and (j)(4)(D); and

(ii) The third and fourth sentences of subsection (b)(1) (regarding the filing and publication of patent information); and

(B) Subsections (b)(2)(A), (b)(2)(B), (b)(3), and (c)(3) if the investigations relied upon by the applicant for approval of the application were not conducted by or for the applicant and for which the applicant has not obtained a right of reference or use from the person by or for whom the investigations were conducted.

(3) PUBLICATION.—For purposes of this section, the Secretary is authorized to make available to the public the established name of each antibiotic drug that was the subject of any application for marketing received by the Secretary for Health and Human Services under section 507 of the Federal Food, Drug, and Cosmetic Act (21 U.S.C. 357) before the date of enactment of this Act.

(e) DEFINITION.—Section 201 (21 U.S.C. 321), as amended by section 121(a)(1), is further amended by adding at the end the following:

"(jj) The term 'antibiotic drug' means any drug (except drugs for use in animals other than humans) composed wholly or partly of any kind of penicillin, streptomycin, chlortetracycline, chloramphenicol, bacitracin, or any other drug intended for human use containing any quantity of any chemical substance which is produced by a micro-organism and which has the capacity to inhibit or destroy micro-organisms in dilute solution (including a chemically synthesized equivalent of any such substance) or any derivative thereof.".

SEC. 126. ELIMINATION OF CERTAIN LABELING REQUIREMENTS.

(a) PRESCRIPTION DRUGS.—Section 503(b)(4) (21 U.S.C. 353(b)(4)) is amended to read as follows:

"(4)(A) A drug that is subject to paragraph (1) shall be deemed to be misbranded if at any time prior to dispensing the label of the drug fails to bear, at a minimum, the symbol 'Rx only'.

"(B) A drug to which paragraph (1) does not apply shall be deemed to be misbranded if at any time prior to dispensing the label of the drug bears the symbol described in subparagraph (A).".

(b) MISBRANDED DRUG.—Section 502(d) (21 U.S.C. 352(d)) is repealed.

(c) CONFORMING AMENDMENTS.—

(1) Section 503(b)(1) (21 U.S.C. 353(b)(1)) is amended—

(A) by striking subparagraph (A); and

(B) by redesignating subparagraphs (B) and (C) as subparagraphs (A) and (B), respectively.

(2) Section 503(b)(3) (21 U.S.C. 353(b)(3)) is amended by striking "section 502(d) and".

(3) Section 102(9)(A) of the Controlled Substances Act (21 U.S.C. 802(9)(A)) is amended—

(A) in clause (i), by striking "(i)"; and

(B) by striking "(ii)" and all that follows.

SEC. 127. APPLICATION OF FEDERAL LAW TO PRACTICE OF PHARMACY COMPOUNDING.

(a) AMENDMENT.—Chapter V is amended by inserting after section 503 (21 U.S.C. 353) the following:

21 USC 353a.

"SEC. 503A. PHARMACY COMPOUNDING.

"(a) IN GENERAL.—Sections 501(a)(2)(B), 502(f)(1), and 505 shall not apply to a drug product if the drug product is compounded for an identified individual patient based on the unsolicited receipt of a valid prescription order or a notation, approved by the prescribing practitioner, on the prescription order that a compounded product is necessary for the identified patient, if the drug product meets the requirements of this section, and if the compounding—

"(1) is by—

"(A) a licensed pharmacist in a State licensed pharmacy or a Federal facility, or

"(B) a licensed physician,

on the prescription order for such individual patient made by a licensed physician or other licensed practitioner authorized by State law to prescribe drugs; or

"(2)(A) is by a licensed pharmacist or licensed physician in limited quantities before the receipt of a valid prescription order for such individual patient; and

"(B) is based on a history of the licensed pharmacist or licensed physician receiving valid prescription orders for the compounding of the drug product, which orders have been generated solely within an established relationship between—

"(i) the licensed pharmacist or licensed physician; and

"(ii)(I) such individual patient for whom the prescription order will be provided; or

"(II) the physician or other licensed practitioner who will write such prescription order.

"(b) COMPOUNDED DRUG.—

"(1) LICENSED PHARMACIST AND LICENSED PHYSICIAN.—A drug product may be compounded under subsection (a) if the licensed pharmacist or licensed physician—

"(A) compounds the drug product using bulk drug substances, as defined in regulations of the Secretary published at section 207.3(a)(4) of title 21 of the Code of Federal Regulations—

"(i) that—

"(I) comply with the standards of an applicable United States Pharmacopoeia or National Formulary monograph, if a monograph exists, and the United States Pharmacopoeia chapter on pharmacy compounding;

"(II) if such a monograph does not exist, are drug substances that are components of drugs approved by the Secretary; or

"(III) if such a monograph does not exist and the drug substance is not a component of a drug approved by the Secretary, that appear on a list developed by the Secretary through regulations issued by the Secretary under subsection (d);

"(ii) that are manufactured by an establishment that is registered under section 510 (including a foreign establishment that is registered under section 510(i)); and

"(iii) that are accompanied by valid certificates of analysis for each bulk drug substance;

"(B) compounds the drug product using ingredients (other than bulk drug substances) that comply with the standards of an applicable United States Pharmacopoeia or National Formulary monograph, if a monograph exists, and the United States Pharmacopoeia chapter on pharmacy compounding;

"(C) does not compound a drug product that appears on a list published by the Secretary in the Federal Register of drug products that have been withdrawn or removed from the market because such drug products or components of such drug products have been found to be unsafe or not effective; and

"(D) does not compound regularly or in inordinate amounts (as defined by the Secretary) any drug products that are essentially copies of a commercially available drug product.

"(2) DEFINITION.—For purposes of paragraph (1)(D), the term 'essentially a copy of a commercially available drug product' does not include a drug product in which there is a change, made for an identified individual patient, which produces for that patient a significant difference, as determined by the prescribing practitioner, between the compounded drug and the comparable commercially available drug product.

"(3) DRUG PRODUCT.—A drug product may be compounded under subsection (a) only if—

"(A) such drug product is not a drug product identified by the Secretary by regulation as a drug product that presents demonstrable difficulties for compounding that reasonably demonstrate an adverse effect on the safety or effectiveness of that drug product; and

"(B) such drug product is compounded in a State—

"(i) that has entered into a memorandum of understanding with the Secretary which addresses the distribution of inordinate amounts of compounded drug products interstate and provides for appropriate investigation by a State agency of complaints relating to compounded drug products distributed outside such State; or

"(ii) that has not entered into the memorandum of understanding described in clause (i) and the licensed pharmacist, licensed pharmacy, or licensed physician distributes (or causes to be distributed) compounded drug products out of the State in which they are compounded in quantities that do not exceed 5 percent of the total prescription orders dispensed or distributed by such pharmacy or physician.

The Secretary shall, in consultation with the National Association of Boards of Pharmacy, develop a standard memorandum of understanding for use by the States in complying with subparagraph (B)(i).

"(c) ADVERTISING AND PROMOTION.—A drug may be compounded under subsection (a) only if the pharmacy, licensed pharmacist, or licensed physician does not advertise or promote the compounding of any particular drug, class of drug, or type of drug. The pharmacy, licensed pharmacist, or licensed physician may advertise and promote the compounding service provided by the licensed pharmacist or licensed physician.

"(d) REGULATIONS.—

"(1) IN GENERAL.—The Secretary shall issue regulations to implement this section. Before issuing regulations to implement subsections (b)(1)(A)(i)(III), (b)(1)(C), or (b)(3)(A), the Secretary shall convene and consult an advisory committee on compounding unless the Secretary determines that the issuance of such regulations before consultation is necessary to protect the public health. The advisory committee shall include representatives from the National Association of Boards of Pharmacy, the United States Pharmacopoeia, pharmacy, physician, and consumer organizations, and other experts selected by the Secretary.

"(2) LIMITING COMPOUNDING.—The Secretary, in consultation with the United States Pharmacopoeia Convention, Incorporated, shall promulgate regulations identifying drug substances that may be used in compounding under subsection (b)(1)(A)(i)(III) for which a monograph does not exist or which are not components of drug products approved by the Secretary. The Secretary shall include in the regulation the criteria for such substances, which shall include historical use, reports in peer reviewed medical literature, or other criteria the Secretary may identify.

"(e) APPLICATION.—This section shall not apply to—

"(1) compounded positron emission tomography drugs as defined in section 201(ii); or

"(2) radiopharmaceuticals.

"(f) DEFINITION.—As used in this section, the term 'compounding' does not include mixing, reconstituting, or other such acts that are performed in accordance with directions contained in approved labeling provided by the product's manufacturer and other manufacturer directions consistent with that labeling.".

21 USC 353a note.

(b) EFFECTIVE DATE.—Section 503A of the Federal Food, Drug, and Cosmetic Act, added by subsection (a), shall take effect upon the expiration of the 1-year period beginning on the date of the enactment of this Act.

SEC. 128. REAUTHORIZATION OF CLINICAL PHARMACOLOGY PROGRAM.

Section 2 of Public Law 102–222 (105 Stat. 1677) is amended—

(1) in subsection (a), by striking "a grant" and all that follows through "Such grant" and inserting the following: "grants for a pilot program for the training of individuals in clinical pharmacology at appropriate medical schools. Such grants"; and

(2) in subsection (b), by striking "to carry out this section" and inserting ", and for fiscal years 1998 through 2002 $3,000,000 for each fiscal year, to carry out this section".

SEC. 129. REGULATIONS FOR SUNSCREEN PRODUCTS.

21 USC 393 note.

Not later than 18 months after the date of enactment of this Act, the Secretary of Health and Human Services shall issue regulations for over-the-counter sunscreen products for the prevention or treatment of sunburn.

SEC. 130. REPORTS OF POSTMARKETING APPROVAL STUDIES.

(a) IN GENERAL.—Chapter V, as amended by section 116, is further amended by inserting after section 506A the following:

"SEC. 506B. REPORTS OF POSTMARKETING STUDIES.

21 USC 356b.

"(a) SUBMISSION.—

"(1) IN GENERAL.—A sponsor of a drug that has entered into an agreement with the Secretary to conduct a postmarketing study of a drug shall submit to the Secretary, within 1 year after the approval of such drug and annually thereafter until the study is completed or terminated, a report of the progress of the study or the reasons for the failure of the sponsor to conduct the study. The report shall be submitted in such form as is prescribed by the Secretary in regulations issued by the Secretary.

"(2) AGREEMENTS PRIOR TO EFFECTIVE DATE.—Any agreement entered into between the Secretary and a sponsor of a drug, prior to the date of enactment of the Food and Drug Administration Modernization Act of 1997, to conduct a postmarketing study of a drug shall be subject to the requirements of paragraph (1). An initial report for such an agreement shall be submitted within 6 months after the date of the issuance of the regulations under paragraph (1).

"(b) CONSIDERATION OF INFORMATION AS PUBLIC INFORMATION.—Any information pertaining to a report described in subsection (a) shall be considered to be public information to the extent that the information is necessary—

"(1) to identify the sponsor; and

"(2) to establish the status of a study described in subsection (a) and the reasons, if any, for any failure to carry out the study.

"(c) STATUS OF STUDIES AND REPORTS.—The Secretary shall annually develop and publish in the Federal Register a report that provides information on the status of the postmarketing studies—

Federal Register, publication.

"(1) that sponsors have entered into agreements to conduct; and

"(2) for which reports have been submitted under subsection (a)(1).".

(b) REPORT TO CONGRESSIONAL COMMITTEES.—Not later than October 1, 2001, the Secretary shall prepare and submit to the Committee on Labor and Human Resources of the Senate and the Committee on Commerce of the House of Representatives a report containing—

21 USC 356b note.

(1) a summary of the reports submitted under section 506B of the Federal Food, Drug, and Cosmetic Act;

(2) an evaluation of—

(A) the performance of the sponsors referred to in such section in fulfilling the agreements with respect to the conduct of postmarketing studies described in such section of such Act; and

(B) the timeliness of the Secretary's review of the postmarketing studies; and

(3) any legislative recommendations respecting the postmarketing studies.

SEC. 131. NOTIFICATION OF DISCONTINUANCE OF A LIFE SAVING PRODUCT.

(a) IN GENERAL.—Chapter V, as amended by section 130, is further amended by inserting after section 506B the following:

21 USC 356c.

"SEC. 506C. DISCONTINUANCE OF A LIFE SAVING PRODUCT.

"(a) IN GENERAL.—A manufacturer that is the sole manufacturer of a drug—

"(1) that is—

"(A) life-supporting;

"(B) life-sustaining; or

"(C) intended for use in the prevention of a debilitating disease or condition;

"(2) for which an application has been approved under section 505(b) or 505(j); and

"(3) that is not a product that was originally derived from human tissue and was replaced by a recombinant product, shall notify the Secretary of a discontinuance of the manufacture of the drug at least 6 months prior to the date of the discontinuance.

"(b) REDUCTION IN NOTIFICATION PERIOD.—The notification period required under subsection (a) for a manufacturer may be reduced if the manufacturer certifies to the Secretary that good cause exists for the reduction, such as a situation in which—

"(1) a public health problem may result from continuation of the manufacturing for the 6-month period;

"(2) a biomaterials shortage prevents the continuation of the manufacturing for the 6-month period;

"(3) a liability problem may exist for the manufacturer if the manufacturing is continued for the 6-month period;

"(4) continuation of the manufacturing for the 6-month period may cause substantial economic hardship for the manufacturer;

"(5) the manufacturer has filed for bankruptcy under chapter 7 or 11 of title 11, United States Code; or

"(6) the manufacturer can continue the distribution of the drug involved for 6 months.

"(c) DISTRIBUTION.—To the maximum extent practicable, the Secretary shall distribute information on the discontinuation of the drugs described in subsection (a) to appropriate physician and patient organizations.".

TITLE II—IMPROVING REGULATION OF DEVICES

SEC. 201. INVESTIGATIONAL DEVICE EXEMPTIONS.

(a) IN GENERAL.—Section 520(g) (21 U.S.C. 360j(g)) is amended by adding at the end the following:

"(6)(A) Not later than 1 year after the date of the enactment of the Food and Drug Administration Modernization Act of 1997, the Secretary shall by regulation establish, with respect to a device for which an exemption under this subsection is in effect, procedures and conditions that, without requiring an additional approval of an application for an exemption or the approval of a supplement to such an application, permit—

"(i) developmental changes in the device (including manufacturing changes) that do not constitute a significant change in design or in basic principles of operation and that are made in response to information gathered during the course of an investigation; and

"(ii) changes or modifications to clinical protocols that do not affect—

"(I) the validity of data or information resulting from the completion of an approved protocol, or the relationship of likely patient risk to benefit relied upon to approve a protocol;

"(II) the scientific soundness of an investigational plan submitted under paragraph (3)(A); or

"(III) the rights, safety, or welfare of the human subjects involved in the investigation.

"(B) Regulations under subparagraph (A) shall provide that a change or modification described in such subparagraph may be made if—

"(i) the sponsor of the investigation determines, on the basis of credible information (as defined by the Secretary) that the applicable conditions under subparagraph (A) are met; and

"(ii) the sponsor submits to the Secretary, not later than 5 days after making the change or modification, a notice of the change or modification.

"(7)(A) In the case of a person intending to investigate the safety or effectiveness of a class III device or any implantable device, the Secretary shall ensure that the person has an opportunity, prior to submitting an application to the Secretary or to an institutional review committee, to submit to the Secretary, for review, an investigational plan (including a clinical protocol). If the applicant submits a written request for a meeting with the Secretary regarding such review, the Secretary shall, not later than 30 days after receiving the request, meet with the applicant for the purpose of reaching agreement regarding the investigational plan (including a clinical protocol). The written request shall include a detailed description of the device, a detailed description of the proposed conditions of use of the device, a proposed plan (including a clinical protocol) for determining whether there is a reasonable assurance of effectiveness, and, if available, information regarding the expected performance from the device.

"(B) Any agreement regarding the parameters of an investigational plan (including a clinical protocol) that is reached between the Secretary and a sponsor or applicant shall be reduced to writing and made part of the administrative record by the Secretary. Any such agreement shall not be changed, except—

"(i) with the written agreement of the sponsor or applicant; or

"(ii) pursuant to a decision, made in accordance with subparagraph (C) by the director of the office in which the device involved is reviewed, that a substantial scientific issue essential to determining the safety or effectiveness of the device involved has been identified.

"(C) A decision under subparagraph (B)(ii) by the director shall be in writing, and may be made only after the Secretary has provided to the sponsor or applicant an opportunity for a meeting at which the director and the sponsor or applicant are present and at which the director documents the scientific issue involved.".

(b) ACTION ON APPLICATION.—Section 515(d)(1)(B) (21 U.S.C. 360e(d)(1)(B)) is amended by adding at the end the following:

"(iii) The Secretary shall accept and review statistically valid and reliable data and any other information from investigations conducted under the authority of regulations required by section 520(g) to make a determination of whether there is a reasonable assurance of safety and effectiveness of a device subject to a pending application under this section if—

"(I) the data or information is derived from investigations of an earlier version of the device, the device has been modified during or after the investigations (but prior to submission of an application under subsection (c)) and such a modification of the device does not constitute a significant change in the design or in the basic principles of operation of the device that would invalidate the data or information; or

"(II) the data or information relates to a device approved under this section, is available for use under this Act, and is relevant to the design and intended use of the device for which the application is pending.".

SEC. 202. SPECIAL REVIEW FOR CERTAIN DEVICES.

Section 515(d) (21 U.S.C. 360e(d)) is amended—
    (1) by redesignating paragraph (3) as paragraph (4); and
    (2) by adding at the end the following:

"(5) In order to provide for more effective treatment or diagnosis of life-threatening or irreversibly debilitating human diseases or conditions, the Secretary shall provide review priority for devices—
    "(A) representing breakthrough technologies,
    "(B) for which no approved alternatives exist,
    "(C) which offer significant advantages over existing approved alternatives, or
    "(D) the availability of which is in the best interest of the patients.".

SEC. 203. EXPANDING HUMANITARIAN USE OF DEVICES.

Section 520(m) (21 U.S.C. 360j(m)) is amended—
    (1) in paragraph (2), by adding after and below subparagraph (C) the following sentences:
"The request shall be in the form of an application submitted to the Secretary. Not later than 75 days after the date of the receipt of the application, the Secretary shall issue an order approving or denying the application.";
    (2) in paragraph (4)—
        (A) in subparagraph (B), by inserting after "(2)(A)" the following: ", unless a physician determines in an emergency situation that approval from a local institutional review committee can not be obtained in time to prevent serious harm or death to a patient"; and
        (B) by adding after and below subparagraph (B) the following:

"In a case described in subparagraph (B) in which a physician uses a device without an approval from an institutional review committee, the physician shall, after the use of the device, notify the chairperson of the local institutional review committee of such use. Such notification shall include the identification of the patient involved, the date on which the device was used, and the reason for the use.";

(3) by amending paragraph (5) to read as follows:

"(5) The Secretary may require a person granted an exemption under paragraph (2) to demonstrate continued compliance with the requirements of this subsection if the Secretary believes such demonstration to be necessary to protect the public health or if the Secretary has reason to believe that the criteria for the exemption are no longer met."; and

(4) by amending paragraph (6) to read as follows:

"(6) The Secretary may suspend or withdraw an exemption from the effectiveness requirements of sections 514 and 515 for a humanitarian device only after providing notice and an opportunity for an informal hearing.".

SEC. 204. DEVICE STANDARDS.

(a) ALTERNATIVE PROCEDURE.—Section 514 (21 U.S.C. 360d) is amended by adding at the end the following:

"Recognition of a Standard

"(c)(1)(A) In addition to establishing a performance standard under this section, the Secretary shall, by publication in the Federal Register, recognize all or part of an appropriate standard established by a nationally or internationally recognized standard development organization for which a person may submit a declaration of conformity in order to meet a premarket submission requirement or other requirement under this Act to which such standard is applicable.

"(B) If a person elects to use a standard recognized by the Secretary under subparagraph (A) to meet the requirements described in such subparagraph, the person shall provide a declaration of conformity to the Secretary that certifies that the device is in conformity with such standard. A person may elect to use data, or information, other than data required by a standard recognized under subparagraph (A) to meet any requirement regarding devices under this Act.

"(2) The Secretary may withdraw such recognition of a standard through publication of a notice in the Federal Register if the Secretary determines that the standard is no longer appropriate for meeting a requirement regarding devices under this Act.

"(3)(A) Subject to subparagraph (B), the Secretary shall accept a declaration of conformity that a device is in conformity with a standard recognized under paragraph (1) unless the Secretary finds—

"(i) that the data or information submitted to support such declaration does not demonstrate that the device is in conformity with the standard identified in the declaration of conformity; or

"(ii) that the standard identified in the declaration of conformity is not applicable to the particular device under review.

Federal Register, publication.

Federal Register, publication.

"(B) The Secretary may request, at any time, the data or information relied on by the person to make a declaration of conformity with respect to a standard recognized under paragraph (1).

"(C) A person making a declaration of conformity with respect to a standard recognized under paragraph (1) shall maintain the data and information demonstrating conformity of the device to the standard for a period of two years after the date of the classification or approval of the device by the Secretary or a period equal to the expected design life of the device, whichever is longer.".

(b) SECTION 301.—Section 301 (21 U.S.C. 331) is amended by adding at the end the following:

"(x) The falsification of a declaration of conformity submitted under section 514(c) or the failure or refusal to provide data or information requested by the Secretary under paragraph (3) of such section.".

(c) SECTION 501.—Section 501(e) (21 U.S.C. 351(e)) is amended—

(1) by striking "(e)" and inserting "(e)(1)"; and

(2) by inserting at the end the following:

"(2) If it is declared to be, purports to be, or is represented as, a device that is in conformity with any standard recognized under section 514(c) unless such device is in all respects in conformity with such standard.".

(d) CONFORMING AMENDMENTS.—Section 514(a) (21 U.S.C. 360d(a)) is amended—

(1) in paragraph (1), in the second sentence, by striking "under this section" and inserting "under subsection (b)";

(2) in paragraph (2), in the matter preceding subparagraph (A), by striking "under this section" and inserting "under subsection (b)";

(3) in paragraph (3), by striking "under this section" and inserting "under subsection (b)"; and

(4) in paragraph (4), in the matter preceding subparagraph (A), by striking "this section" and inserting "this subsection and subsection (b)".

SEC. 205. SCOPE OF REVIEW; COLLABORATIVE DETERMINATIONS OF DEVICE DATA REQUIREMENTS.

(a) SECTION 513(a).—Section 513(a)(3) (21 U.S.C. 360c(a)(3)) is amended by adding at the end the following:

"(C) In making a determination of a reasonable assurance of the effectiveness of a device for which an application under section 515 has been submitted, the Secretary shall consider whether the extent of data that otherwise would be required for approval of the application with respect to effectiveness can be reduced through reliance on postmarket controls.

"(D)(i) The Secretary, upon the written request of any person intending to submit an application under section 515, shall meet with such person to determine the type of valid scientific evidence (within the meaning of subparagraphs (A) and (B)) that will be necessary to demonstrate for purposes of approval of an application the effectiveness of a device for the conditions of use proposed by such person. The written request shall include a detailed description of the device, a detailed description of the proposed conditions of use of the device, a proposed plan for determining whether there is a reasonable assurance of effectiveness, and, if available, information regarding the expected performance from the device. Within 30 days after such meeting, the Secretary shall specify in writing the type of valid scientific evidence that will provide a reasonable assurance that a device is effective under the conditions of use proposed by such person.

"(ii) Any clinical data, including one or more well-controlled investigations, specified in writing by the Secretary for demonstrating a reasonable assurance of device effectiveness shall be specified as result of a determination by the Secretary that such data are necessary to establish device effectiveness. The Secretary shall consider, in consultation with the applicant, the least burdensome appropriate means of evaluating device effectiveness that would have a reasonable likelihood of resulting in approval.

"(iii) The determination of the Secretary with respect to the specification of valid scientific evidence under clauses (i) and (ii) shall be binding upon the Secretary, unless such determination by the Secretary could be contrary to the public health.".

(b) SECTION 513(i).—Section 513(i)(1) (21 U.S.C. 360c(i)(1)) is amended by adding at the end the following:

"(C) To facilitate reviews of reports submitted to the Secretary under section 510(k), the Secretary shall consider the extent to which reliance on postmarket controls may expedite the classification of devices under subsection (f)(1) of this section.

"(D) Whenever the Secretary requests information to demonstrate that devices with differing technological characteristics are substantially equivalent, the Secretary shall only request information that is necessary to making substantial equivalence determinations. In making such request, the Secretary shall consider the least burdensome means of demonstrating substantial equivalence and request information accordingly.

"(E)(i) Any determination by the Secretary of the intended use of a device shall be based upon the proposed labeling submitted in a report for the device under section 510(k). However, when determining that a device can be found substantially equivalent to a legally marketed device, the director of the organizational unit responsible for regulating devices (in this subparagraph referred to as the 'Director') may require a statement in labeling that provides appropriate information regarding a use of the device not identified in the proposed labeling if, after providing an opportunity for consultation with the person who submitted such report, the Director determines and states in writing—

"(I) that there is a reasonable likelihood that the device will be used for an intended use not identified in the proposed labeling for the device; and

"(II) that such use could cause harm.

"(ii) Such determination shall—

"(I) be provided to the person who submitted the report within 10 days from the date of the notification of the Director's concerns regarding the proposed labeling;

"(II) specify the limitations on the use of the device not included in the proposed labeling; and

"(III) find the device substantially equivalent if the requirements of subparagraph (A) are met and if the labeling for such device conforms to the limitations specified in subclause (II).

"(iii) The responsibilities of the Director under this subparagraph may not be delegated.

"(iv) This subparagraph has no legal effect after the expiration of the five-year period beginning on the date of the enactment of the Food and Drug Administration Modernization Act of 1997.".

(c) SECTION 515(d).—Section 515(d) (21 U.S.C. 360e(d)) is amended—

(1) in paragraph (1)(A), by adding after and below clause (ii) the following:

"In making the determination whether to approve or deny the application, the Secretary shall rely on the conditions of use included in the proposed labeling as the basis for determining whether or not there is a reasonable assurance of safety and effectiveness, if the proposed labeling is neither false nor misleading. In determining whether or not such labeling is false or misleading, the Secretary shall fairly evaluate all material facts pertinent to the proposed labeling."; and

(2) by adding after paragraph (5) (as added by section 202(2)) the following:

"(6)(A)(i) A supplemental application shall be required for any change to a device subject to an approved application under this subsection that affects safety or effectiveness, unless such change is a modification in a manufacturing procedure or method of manufacturing and the holder of the approved application submits a written notice to the Secretary that describes in detail the change, summarizes the data or information supporting the change, and informs the Secretary that the change has been made under the requirements of section 520(f).

"(ii) The holder of an approved application who submits a notice under clause (i) with respect to a manufacturing change of a device may distribute the device 30 days after the date on which the Secretary receives the notice, unless the Secretary within such 30-day period notifies the holder that the notice is not adequate and describes such further information or action that is required for acceptance of such change. If the Secretary notifies the holder that a supplemental application is required, the Secretary shall review the supplement within 135 days after the receipt of the supplement. The time used by the Secretary to review the notice of the manufacturing change shall be deducted from the 135-day review period if the notice meets appropriate content requirements for premarket approval supplements.

"(B)(i) Subject to clause (ii), in reviewing a supplement to an approved application, for an incremental change to the design of a device that affects safety or effectiveness, the Secretary shall approve such supplement if—

"(I) nonclinical data demonstrate that the design modification creates the intended additional capacity, function, or performance of the device; and

"(II) clinical data from the approved application and any supplement to the approved application provide a reasonable assurance of safety and effectiveness for the changed device.

"(ii) The Secretary may require, when necessary, additional clinical data to evaluate the design modification of the device to provide a reasonable assurance of safety and effectiveness.".

SEC. 206. PREMARKET NOTIFICATION.

(a) SECTION 510.—Section 510 (21 U.S.C. 360) is amended—

(1) in subsection (k), in the matter preceding paragraph (1), by adding after "report to the Secretary" the following: "or person who is accredited under section 523(a)"; and

(2) by adding at the end the following subsections:

"(l) A report under subsection (k) is not required for a device intended for human use that is exempted from the requirements of this subsection under subsection (m) or is within a type that has been classified into class I under section 513. The exception established in the preceding sentence does not apply to any class I device that is intended for a use which is of substantial importance in preventing impairment of human health, or to any class I device that presents a potential unreasonable risk of illness or injury.

"(m)(1) Not later than 60 days after the date of enactment of the Food and Drug Administration Modernization Act of 1997, the Secretary shall publish in the Federal Register a list of each type of class II device that does not require a report under subsection (k) to provide reasonable assurance of safety and effectiveness. Each type of class II device identified by the Secretary as not requiring the report shall be exempt from the requirement to provide a report under subsection (k) as of the date of the publication of the list in the Federal Register.

Federal Register, publication.

"(2) Beginning on the date that is 1 day after the date of the publication of a list under this subsection, the Secretary may exempt a class II device from the requirement to submit a report under subsection (k), upon the Secretary's own initiative or a petition of an interested person, if the Secretary determines that such report is not necessary to assure the safety and effectiveness of the device. The Secretary shall publish in the Federal Register notice of the intent of the Secretary to exempt the device, or of the petition, and provide a 30-day period for public comment. Within 120 days after the issuance of the notice in the Federal Register, the Secretary shall publish an order in the Federal Register that sets forth the final determination of the Secretary regarding the exemption of the device that was the subject of the notice. If the Secretary fails to respond to a petition within 180 days of receiving it, the petition shall be deemed to be granted.".

Federal Register, publication.

Federal Register, publication.

(b) SECTION 513(f).—Section 513(f) (21 U.S.C. 360c(f)) is amended by adding at the end the following:

"(5) The Secretary may not withhold a determination of the initial classification of a device under paragraph (1) because of a failure to comply with any provision of this Act unrelated to a substantial equivalence decision, including a finding that the facility in which the device is manufactured is not in compliance with good manufacturing requirements as set forth in regulations of the Secretary under section 520(f) (other than a finding that there is a substantial likelihood that the failure to comply with such regulations will potentially present a serious risk to human health).".

(c) SECTION 513(i).—Section 513(i)(1) (21 U.S.C. 360c(i)), as amended by section 205(b), is amended—

(1) in subparagraph (A)(ii)—

(A) in subclause (I), by striking "clinical data" and inserting "appropriate clinical or scientific data" and by inserting "or a person accredited under section 523" after "Secretary"; and

(B) in subclause (II), by striking "efficacy" and inserting "effectiveness"; and

(2) by adding at the end the following:

"(F) Not later than 270 days after the date of the enactment of the Food and Drug Administration Modernization Act of 1997, the Secretary shall issue guidance specifying the general principles that the Secretary will consider in determining when a specific intended use of a device is not reasonably included within a general use of such device for purposes of a determination of substantial equivalence under subsection (f) or section 520(l).".

SEC. 207. EVALUATION OF AUTOMATIC CLASS III DESIGNATION.

Section 513(f) (21 U.S.C. 360c(f)), as amended by section 206(b), is amended—

(1) in paragraph (1)—

(A) in subparagraph (B), by striking "paragraph (2)" and inserting "paragraph (3)"; and

(B) in the last sentence, by striking "paragraph (2)" and inserting "paragraph (2) or (3)";

(2) by redesignating paragraphs (2) and (3) as paragraphs (3) and (4), respectively; and

(3) by inserting after paragraph (1) the following:

"(2)(A) Any person who submits a report under section 510(k) for a type of device that has not been previously classified under this Act, and that is classified into class III under paragraph (1), may request, within 30 days after receiving written notice of such a classification, the Secretary to classify the device under the criteria set forth in subparagraphs (A) through (C) of subsection (a)(1). The person may, in the request, recommend to the Secretary a classification for the device. Any such request shall describe the device and provide detailed information and reasons for the recommended classification.

"(B)(i) Not later than 60 days after the date of the submission of the request under subparagraph (A), the Secretary shall by written order classify the device involved. Such classification shall be the initial classification of the device for purposes of paragraph (1) and any device classified under this paragraph shall be a predicate device for determining substantial equivalence under paragraph (1).

"(ii) A device that remains in class III under this subparagraph shall be deemed to be adulterated within the meaning of section 501(f)(1)(B) until approved under section 515 or exempted from such approval under section 520(g).

Federal Register, publication.

"(C) Within 30 days after the issuance of an order classifying a device under this paragraph, the Secretary shall publish a notice in the Federal Register announcing such classification.".

SEC. 208. CLASSIFICATION PANELS.

Section 513(b) (21 U.S.C. 360c(b)) is amended by adding at the end the following:

"(5) Classification panels covering each type of device shall be scheduled to meet at such times as may be appropriate for the Secretary to meet applicable statutory deadlines.

"(6)(A) Any person whose device is specifically the subject of review by a classification panel shall have—

"(i) the same access to data and information submitted to a classification panel (except for data and information that are not available for public disclosure under section 552 of title 5, United States Code) as the Secretary;

"(ii) the opportunity to submit, for review by a classification panel, information that is based on the data or information provided in the application submitted under section 515 by the person, which information shall be submitted to the Secretary for prompt transmittal to the classification panel; and

"(iii) the same opportunity as the Secretary to participate in meetings of the panel.

"(B) Any meetings of a classification panel shall provide adequate time for initial presentations and for response to any differing views by persons whose devices are specifically the subject of a classification panel review, and shall encourage free and open participation by all interested persons.

"(7) After receiving from a classification panel the conclusions and recommendations of the panel on a matter that the panel has reviewed, the Secretary shall review the conclusions and recommendations, shall make a final decision on the matter in accordance with section 515(d)(2), and shall notify the affected persons of the decision in writing and, if the decision differs from the conclusions and recommendations of the panel, shall include the reasons for the difference.

"(8) A classification panel under this subsection shall not be subject to the annual chartering and annual report requirements of the Federal Advisory Committee Act.".

SEC. 209. CERTAINTY OF REVIEW TIMEFRAMES; COLLABORATIVE REVIEW PROCESS.

(a) CERTAINTY OF REVIEW TIMEFRAMES.—Section 510 (21 U.S.C. 360), as amended by section 206(a)(2), is amended by adding at the end the following subsection:

"(n) The Secretary shall review the report required in subsection (k) and make a determination under section 513(f)(1) not later than 90 days after receiving the report.".

(b) COLLABORATIVE REVIEW PROCESS.—Section 515(d) (21 U.S.C. 360e(d)), as amended by section 202(1), is amended by inserting after paragraph (2) the following:

"(3)(A)(i) The Secretary shall, upon the written request of an applicant, meet with the applicant, not later than 100 days after the receipt of an application that has been filed as complete under subsection (c), to discuss the review status of the application.

"(ii) The Secretary shall, in writing and prior to the meeting, provide to the applicant a description of any deficiencies in the application that, at that point, have been identified by the Secretary based on an interim review of the entire application and identify the information that is required to correct those deficiencies.

"(iii) The Secretary shall notify the applicant promptly of—

"(I) any additional deficiency identified in the application, or

"(II) any additional information required to achieve completion of the review and final action on the application,

that was not described as a deficiency in the written description provided by the Secretary under clause (ii).

"(B) The Secretary and the applicant may, by mutual consent, establish a different schedule for a meeting required under this paragraph.

SEC. 210. ACCREDITATION OF PERSONS FOR REVIEW OF PREMARKET NOTIFICATION REPORTS.

(a) IN GENERAL.—Subchapter A of chapter V is amended by adding at the end the following:

21 USC 360m.

"SEC. 523. ACCREDITED PERSONS.

"(a) IN GENERAL.—

"(1) REVIEW AND CLASSIFICATION OF DEVICES.—Not later than 1 year after the date of the enactment of the Food and Drug Administration Modernization Act of 1997, the Secretary shall, subject to paragraph (3), accredit persons for the purpose of reviewing reports submitted under section 510(k) and making recommendations to the Secretary regarding the initial classification of devices under section 513(f)(1).

"(2) REQUIREMENTS REGARDING REVIEW.—

"(A) IN GENERAL.—In making a recommendation to the Secretary under paragraph (1), an accredited person shall notify the Secretary in writing of the reasons for the recommendation.

"(B) TIME PERIOD FOR REVIEW.—Not later than 30 days after the date on which the Secretary is notified under subparagraph (A) by an accredited person with respect to a recommendation of an initial classification of a device, the Secretary shall make a determination with respect to the initial classification.

"(C) SPECIAL RULE.—The Secretary may change the initial classification under section 513(f)(1) that is recommended under paragraph (1) by an accredited person, and in such case shall provide to such person, and the person who submitted the report under section 510(k) for the device, a statement explaining in detail the reasons for the change.

"(3) CERTAIN DEVICES.—

"(A) IN GENERAL.—An accredited person may not be used to perform a review of—

"(i) a class III device;

"(ii) a class II device which is intended to be permanently implantable or life sustaining or life supporting; or

"(iii) a class II device which requires clinical data in the report submitted under section 510(k) for the device, except that the number of class II devices to which the Secretary applies this clause for a year, less the number of such reports to which clauses (i) and (ii) apply, may not exceed 6 percent of the number that is equal to the total number of reports submitted to the Secretary under such section for such year less the number of such reports to which such clauses apply for such year.

"(B) ADJUSTMENT.—In determining for a year the ratio described in subparagraph (A)(iii), the Secretary shall not include in the numerator class III devices that the Secretary reclassified into class II, and the Secretary shall include in the denominator class II devices for which reports under section 510(k) were not required to be submitted by reason of the operation of section 510(m).

"(b) ACCREDITATION.—

"(1) PROGRAMS.—The Secretary shall provide for such accreditation through programs administered by the Food and Drug Administration, other government agencies, or by other qualified nongovernment organizations.

"(2) ACCREDITATION.—

"(A) IN GENERAL.—Not later than 180 days after the date of the enactment of the Food and Drug Administration Modernization Act of 1997, the Secretary shall establish and publish in the Federal Register criteria to accredit or deny accreditation to persons who request to perform the duties specified in subsection (a). The Secretary shall respond to a request for accreditation within 60 days of the receipt of the request. The accreditation of such person shall specify the particular activities under subsection (a) for which such person is accredited.

Federal Register, publication.

"(B) WITHDRAWAL OF ACCREDITATION.—The Secretary may suspend or withdraw accreditation of any person accredited under this paragraph, after providing notice and an opportunity for an informal hearing, when such person is substantially not in compliance with the requirements of this section or poses a threat to public health or fails to act in a manner that is consistent with the purposes of this section.

"(C) PERFORMANCE AUDITING.—To ensure that persons accredited under this section will continue to meet the standards of accreditation, the Secretary shall—

"(i) make onsite visits on a periodic basis to each accredited person to audit the performance of such person; and

"(ii) take such additional measures as the Secretary determines to be appropriate.

"(D) ANNUAL REPORT.—The Secretary shall include in the annual report required under section 903(g) the names of all accredited persons and the particular activities under subsection (a) for which each such person is accredited and the name of each accredited person whose accreditation has been withdrawn during the year.

"(3) QUALIFICATIONS.—An accredited person shall, at a minimum, meet the following requirements:

"(A) Such person may not be an employee of the Federal Government.

"(B) Such person shall be an independent organization which is not owned or controlled by a manufacturer, supplier, or vendor of devices and which has no organizational, material, or financial affiliation with such a manufacturer, supplier, or vendor.

"(C) Such person shall be a legally constituted entity permitted to conduct the activities for which it seeks accreditation.

"(D) Such person shall not engage in the design, manufacture, promotion, or sale of devices.

"(E) The operations of such person shall be in accordance with generally accepted professional and ethical business practices and shall agree in writing that as a minimum it will—

"(i) certify that reported information accurately reflects data reviewed;

66

"(ii) limit work to that for which competence and capacity are available;

"(iii) treat information received, records, reports, and recommendations as proprietary information;

"(iv) promptly respond and attempt to resolve complaints regarding its activities for which it is accredited; and

"(v) protect against the use, in carrying out subsection (a) with respect to a device, of any officer or employee of the person who has a financial conflict of interest regarding the device, and annually make available to the public disclosures of the extent to which the person, and the officers and employees of the person, have maintained compliance with requirements under this clause relating to financial conflicts of interest.

"(4) SELECTION OF ACCREDITED PERSONS.—The Secretary shall provide each person who chooses to use an accredited person to receive a section 510(k) report a panel of at least two or more accredited persons from which the regulated person may select one for a specific regulatory function.

"(5) COMPENSATION OF ACCREDITED PERSONS.—Compensation for an accredited person shall be determined by agreement between the accredited person and the person who engages the services of the accredited person, and shall be paid by the person who engages such services.

"(c) DURATION.—The authority provided by this section terminates—

"(1) 5 years after the date on which the Secretary notifies Congress that at least 2 persons accredited under subsection (b) are available to review at least 60 percent of the submissions under section 510(k), or

"(2) 4 years after the date on which the Secretary notifies Congress that the Secretary has made a determination described in paragraph (2)(B) of subsection (a) for at least 35 percent of the devices that are subject to review under paragraph (1) of such subsection,

whichever occurs first.".

(b) RECORDKEEPING.—Section 704 (21 U.S.C. 374) is amended by adding at the end the following:

"(f)(1) A person accredited under section 523 to review reports made under section 510(k) and make recommendations of initial classifications of devices to the Secretary shall maintain records documenting the training qualifications of the person and the employees of the person, the procedures used by the person for handling confidential information, the compensation arrangements made by the person, and the procedures used by the person to identify and avoid conflicts of interest. Upon the request of an officer or employee designated by the Secretary, the person shall permit the officer or employee, at all reasonable times, to have access to, to copy, and to verify, the records.

"(2) Within 15 days after the receipt of a written request from the Secretary to a person accredited under section 523 for copies of records described in paragraph (1), the person shall produce the copies of the records at the place designated by the Secretary.".

(c) CONFORMING AMENDMENT.—Section 301 (21 U.S.C. 331), as amended by section 204(b), is amended by adding at the end the following:

"(y) In the case of a drug, device, or food—

"(1) the submission of a report or recommendation by a person accredited under section 523 that is false or misleading in any material respect;

"(2) the disclosure by a person accredited under section 523 of confidential commercial information or any trade secret without the express written consent of the person who submitted such information or secret to such person; or

"(3) the receipt by a person accredited under section 523 of a bribe in any form or the doing of any corrupt act by such person associated with a responsibility delegated to such person under this Act.".

(d) REPORTS ON PROGRAM OF ACCREDITATION.—

21 USC 360m note.

(1) COMPTROLLER GENERAL.—

(A) IMPLEMENTATION OF PROGRAM.—Not later than 5 years after the date of the enactment of this Act, the Comptroller General of the United States shall submit to the Committee on Commerce of the House of Representatives and the Committee on Labor and Human Resources of the Senate a report describing the extent to which the program of accreditation required by the amendment made by subsection (a) has been implemented.

(B) EVALUATION OF PROGRAM.—Not later than 6 months prior to the date on which, pursuant to subsection (c) of section 523 of the Federal Food, Drug, and Cosmetic Act (as added by subsection (a)), the authority provided under subsection (a) of such section will terminate, the Comptroller General shall submit to the Committee on Commerce of the House of Representatives and the Committee on Labor and Human Resources of the Senate a report describing the use of accredited persons under such section 523, including an evaluation of the extent to which such use assisted the Secretary in carrying out the duties of the Secretary under such Act with respect to devices, and the extent to which such use promoted actions which are contrary to the purposes of such Act.

(2) INCLUSION OF CERTAIN DEVICES WITHIN PROGRAM.—Not later than 3 years after the date of the enactment of this Act, the Secretary of Health and Human Services shall submit to the Committee on Commerce of the House of Representatives and the Committee on Labor and Human Resources of the Senate a report providing a determination by the Secretary of whether, in the program of accreditation established pursuant to the amendment made by subsection (a), the limitation established in clause (iii) of section 523(a)(3)(A) of the Federal Food, Drug, and Cosmetic Act (relating to class II devices for which clinical data are required in reports under section 510(k)) should be removed.

SEC. 211. DEVICE TRACKING.

Effective 90 days after the date of the enactment of this Act, section 519(e) (21 U.S.C. 360i(e)) is amended to read as follows:

"Device Tracking

"(e)(1) The Secretary may by order require a manufacturer to adopt a method of tracking a class II or class III device—
    "(A) the failure of which would be reasonably likely to have serious adverse health consequences; or
    "(B) which is—
        "(i) intended to be implanted in the human body for more than one year, or
        "(ii) a life sustaining or life supporting device used outside a device user facility.
"(2) Any patient receiving a device subject to tracking under paragraph (1) may refuse to release, or refuse permission to release, the patient's name, address, social security number, or other identifying information for the purpose of tracking.".

SEC. 212. POSTMARKET SURVEILLANCE.

Effective 90 days after the date of the enactment of this Act, section 522 (21 U.S.C. 360l) is amended to read as follows:

"POSTMARKET SURVEILLANCE

"SEC. 522. (a) IN GENERAL.—The Secretary may by order require a manufacturer to conduct postmarket surveillance for any device of the manufacturer which is a class II or class III device the failure of which would be reasonably likely to have serious adverse health consequences or which is intended to be—
    "(1) implanted in the human body for more than one year, or
    "(2) a life sustaining or life supporting device used outside a device user facility.
"(b) SURVEILLANCE APPROVAL.—Each manufacturer required to conduct a surveillance of a device shall, within 30 days of receiving an order from the Secretary prescribing that the manufacturer is required under this section to conduct such surveillance, submit, for the approval of the Secretary, a plan for the required surveillance. The Secretary, within 60 days of the receipt of such plan, shall determine if the person designated to conduct the surveillance has appropriate qualifications and experience to undertake such surveillance and if the plan will result in the collection of useful data that can reveal unforeseen adverse events or other information necessary to protect the public health. The Secretary, in consultation with the manufacturer, may by order require a prospective surveillance period of up to 36 months. Any determination by the Secretary that a longer period is necessary shall be made by mutual agreement between the Secretary and the manufacturer or, if no agreement can be reached, after the completion of a dispute resolution process as described in section 562.".

SEC. 213. REPORTS.

(a) REPORTS.—Section 519 (21 U.S.C. 360i) is amended—
    (1) in subsection (a)—
        (A) in the matter preceding paragraph (1), by striking "manufacturer, importer, or distributor" and inserting "manufacturer or importer";
        (B) in paragraph (4), by striking "manufacturer, importer, or distributor" and inserting "manufacturer or importer";

(C) in paragraph (7), by adding "and" after the semi-colon at the end;

(D) in paragraph (8)—

(i) by striking "manufacturer, importer, or distributor" each place such term appears and inserting "manufacturer or importer"; and

(ii) by striking the semicolon at the end and inserting a period;

(E) by striking paragraph (9); and

(F) by inserting at the end the following sentence: "The Secretary shall by regulation require distributors to keep records and make such records available to the Secretary upon request. Paragraphs (4) and (8) apply to distributors to the same extent and in the same manner as such paragraphs apply to manufacturers and importers.";

(2) by striking subsection (d); and

(3) in subsection (f), by striking ", importer, or distributor" each place it appears and inserting "or importer".

(b) REGISTRATION.—Section 510(g) (21 U.S.C. 360(g)) is amended—

(1) by redesignating paragraph (4) as paragraph (5);

(2) by inserting after paragraph (3) the following:

"(4) any distributor who acts as a wholesale distributor of devices, and who does not manufacture, repackage, process, or relabel a device; or"; and

(3) by adding at the end the following flush sentence: "In this subsection, the term 'wholesale distributor' means any person (other than the manufacturer or the initial importer) who distributes a device from the original place of manufacture to the person who makes the final delivery or sale of the device to the ultimate consumer or user.".

(c) DEVICE USER FACILITIES.—

(1) IN GENERAL.—Section 519(b) (21 U.S.C. 360i(b)) is amended—

(A) in paragraph (1)(C)—

(i) in the first sentence, by striking "a semi-annual basis" and inserting "an annual basis";

(ii) in the second sentence, by striking "and July 1"; and

(iii) by striking the matter after and below clause (iv); and

(B) in paragraph (2)—

(i) in subparagraph (A), by inserting "or" after the comma at the end;

(ii) in subparagraph (B), by striking ", or" at the end and inserting a period; and

(iii) by striking subparagraph (C).

(2) SENTINEL SYSTEM.—Section 519(b) (21 U.S.C. 360i(b)) is amended—

(A) by redesignating paragraph (5) as paragraph (6); and

(B) by inserting after paragraph (4) the following paragraph:

"(5) With respect to device user facilities:

"(A) The Secretary shall by regulation plan and implement a program under which the Secretary limits user reporting under paragraphs (1) through (4) to a subset of user facilities that constitutes a representative profile of user reports for device deaths and serious illnesses or serious injuries.

"(B) During the period of planning the program under subparagraph (A), paragraphs (1) through (4) continue to apply.

"(C) During the period in which the Secretary is providing for a transition to the full implementation of the program, paragraphs (1) through (4) apply except to the extent that the Secretary determines otherwise.

"(D) On and after the date on which the program is fully implemented, paragraphs (1) through (4) do not apply to a user facility unless the facility is included in the subset referred to in subparagraph (A).

"(E) Not later than 2 years after the date of the enactment of the Food and Drug Administration Modernization Act of 1997, the Secretary shall submit to the Committee on Commerce of the House of Representatives, and to the Committee on Labor and Human Resources of the Senate, a report describing the plan developed by the Secretary under subparagraph (A) and the progress that has been made toward the implementation of the plan.".

SEC. 214. PRACTICE OF MEDICINE.

Chapter IX is amended by adding at the end the following:

21 USC 396.

"SEC. 906. PRACTICE OF MEDICINE.

"Nothing in this Act shall be construed to limit or interfere with the authority of a health care practitioner to prescribe or administer any legally marketed device to a patient for any condition or disease within a legitimate health care practitioner-patient relationship. This section shall not limit any existing authority of the Secretary to establish and enforce restrictions on the sale or distribution, or in the labeling, of a device that are part of a determination of substantial equivalence, established as a condition of approval, or promulgated through regulations. Further, this section shall not change any existing prohibition on the promotion of unapproved uses of legally marketed devices.".

SEC. 215. NONINVASIVE BLOOD GLUCOSE METER.

(a) FINDINGS.—The Congress finds that—

(1) diabetes and its complications are a leading cause of death by disease in America;

(2) diabetes affects approximately 16,000,000 Americans and another 650,000 will be diagnosed in 1997;

(3) the total health care-related costs of diabetes total nearly $100,000,000,000 per year;

(4) diabetes is a disease that is managed and controlled on a daily basis by the patient;

(5) the failure to properly control and manage diabetes results in costly and often fatal complications including but not limited to blindness, coronary artery disease, and kidney failure;

(6) blood testing devices are a critical tool for the control and management of diabetes, and existing blood testing devices require repeated piercing of the skin;

(7) the pain associated with existing blood testing devices creates a disincentive for people with diabetes to test blood glucose levels, particularly children;

(8) a safe and effective noninvasive blood glucose meter would likely improve control and management of diabetes by increasing the number of tests conducted by people with diabetes, particularly children; and

(9) the Food and Drug Administration is responsible for reviewing all applications for new medical devices in the United States.

(b) SENSE OF CONGRESS.—It is the sense of the Congress that the availability of a safe, effective, noninvasive blood glucose meter would greatly enhance the health and well-being of all people with diabetes across America and the world.

SEC. 216. USE OF DATA RELATING TO PREMARKET APPROVAL; PRODUCT DEVELOPMENT PROTOCOL.

(a) USE OF DATA RELATING TO PREMARKET APPROVAL.—

(1) IN GENERAL.—Section 520(h)(4) (21 U.S.C. 360j(h)(4)) is amended to read as follows:

"(4)(A) Any information contained in an application for premarket approval filed with the Secretary pursuant to section 515(c) (including information from clinical and preclinical tests or studies that demonstrate the safety and effectiveness of a device, but excluding descriptions of methods of manufacture and product composition and other trade secrets) shall be available, 6 years after the application has been approved by the Secretary, for use by the Secretary in—

"(i) approving another device;

"(ii) determining whether a product development protocol has been completed, under section 515 for another device;

"(iii) establishing a performance standard or special control under this Act; or

"(iv) classifying or reclassifying another device under section 513 and subsection (l)(2).

"(B) The publicly available detailed summaries of information respecting the safety and effectiveness of devices required by paragraph (1)(A) shall be available for use by the Secretary as the evidentiary basis for the agency actions described in subparagraph (A).".

(2) CONFORMING AMENDMENTS.—Section 517(a) (21 U.S.C. 360g(a)) is amended—

(A) in paragraph (8), by adding "or" at the end;

(B) in paragraph (9), by striking ", or" and inserting a comma; and

(C) by striking paragraph (10).

(b) PRODUCT DEVELOPMENT PROTOCOL.—Section 515(f)(2) (21 U.S.C. 360e(f)(2)) is amended by striking "he shall" and all that follows and inserting the following: "the Secretary—

"(A) may, at the initiative of the Secretary, refer the proposed protocol to the appropriate panel under section 513 for its recommendation respecting approval of the protocol; or

"(B) shall so refer such protocol upon the request of the submitter, unless the Secretary finds that the proposed protocol and accompanying data which would be reviewed by such panel substantially duplicate a product development protocol and accompanying data which have previously been reviewed by such a panel.".

SEC. 217. CLARIFICATION OF THE NUMBER OF REQUIRED CLINICAL INVESTIGATIONS FOR APPROVAL.

Section 513(a)(3)(A) (21 U.S.C. 360c(a)(3)(A)) is amended by striking "clinical investigations" and inserting "1 or more clinical investigations".

TITLE III—IMPROVING REGULATION OF FOOD

SEC. 301. FLEXIBILITY FOR REGULATIONS REGARDING CLAIMS.

Section 403(r) (21 U.S.C. 343(r)) is amended by adding at the end the following:

"(7) The Secretary may make proposed regulations issued under this paragraph effective upon publication pending consideration of public comment and publication of a final regulation if the Secretary determines that such action is necessary—

"(A) to enable the Secretary to review and act promptly on petitions the Secretary determines provide for information necessary to—

"(i) enable consumers to develop and maintain healthy dietary practices;

"(ii) enable consumers to be informed promptly and effectively of important new knowledge regarding nutritional and health benefits of food; or

"(iii) ensure that scientifically sound nutritional and health information is provided to consumers as soon as possible; or

"(B) to enable the Secretary to act promptly to ban or modify a claim under this paragraph.

Such proposed regulations shall be deemed final agency action for purposes of judicial review.".

SEC. 302. PETITIONS FOR CLAIMS.

Section 403(r)(4)(A)(i) (21 U.S.C. 343(r)(4)(A)(i)) is amended—

(1) by adding after the second sentence the following: "If the Secretary does not act within such 100 days, the petition shall be deemed to be denied unless an extension is mutually agreed upon by the Secretary and the petitioner.";

(2) in the fourth sentence (as amended by paragraph (1)) by inserting immediately before the comma the following: "or the petition is deemed to be denied"; and

(3) by adding at the end the following: "If the Secretary does not act within such 90 days, the petition shall be deemed to be denied unless an extension is mutually agreed upon by the Secretary and the petitioner. If the Secretary issues a proposed regulation, the rulemaking shall be completed within 540 days of the date the petition is received by the Secretary. If the Secretary does not issue a regulation within such 540 days, the Secretary shall provide the Committee on Commerce of the House of Representatives and the Committee on Labor and Human Resources of the Senate the reasons action on the regulation did not occur within such 540 days.".

SEC. 303. HEALTH CLAIMS FOR FOOD PRODUCTS.

Section 403(r)(3) (21 U.S.C. 343(r)(3)) is amended by adding at the end thereof the following:

"(C) Notwithstanding the provisions of clauses (A)(i) and (B), a claim of the type described in subparagraph (1)(B) which is not authorized by the Secretary in a regulation promulgated in accordance with clause (B) shall be authorized and may be made with respect to a food if—

"(i) a scientific body of the United States Government with official responsibility for public health protection or research directly relating to human nutrition (such as the National Institutes of Health or the Centers for Disease Control and Prevention) or the National Academy of Sciences or any of its subdivisions has published an authoritative statement, which is currently in effect, about the relationship between a nutrient and a disease or health-related condition to which the claim refers;

"(ii) a person has submitted to the Secretary, at least 120 days (during which the Secretary may notify any person who is making a claim as authorized by clause (C) that such person has not submitted all the information required by such clause) before the first introduction into interstate commerce of the food with a label containing the claim, (I) a notice of the claim, which shall include the exact words used in the claim and shall include a concise description of the basis upon which such person relied for determining that the requirements of subclause (i) have been satisfied, (II) a copy of the statement referred to in subclause (i) upon which such person relied in making the claim, and (III) a balanced representation of the scientific literature relating to the relationship between a nutrient and a disease or health-related condition to which the claim refers;

"(iii) the claim and the food for which the claim is made are in compliance with clause (A)(ii) and are otherwise in compliance with paragraph (a) and section 201(n); and

"(iv) the claim is stated in a manner so that the claim is an accurate representation of the authoritative statement referred to in subclause (i) and so that the claim enables the public to comprehend the information provided in the claim and to understand the relative significance of such information in the context of a total daily diet.

For purposes of this clause, a statement shall be regarded as an authoritative statement of a scientific body described in subclause (i) only if the statement is published by the scientific body and shall not include a statement of an employee of the scientific body made in the individual capacity of the employee.

"(D) A claim submitted under the requirements of clause (C) may be made until—

"(i) such time as the Secretary issues a regulation under the standard in clause (B)(i)—

"(I) prohibiting or modifying the claim and the regulation has become effective, or

"(II) finding that the requirements of clause (C) have not been met, including finding that the petitioner has not submitted all the information required by such clause; or

"(ii) a district court of the United States in an enforcement proceeding under chapter III has determined that the requirements of clause (C) have not been met.".

SEC. 304. NUTRIENT CONTENT CLAIMS.

Section 403(r)(2) (21 U.S.C. 343(r)(2)) is amended by adding at the end the following:

"(G) A claim of the type described in subparagraph (1)(A) for a nutrient, for which the Secretary has not promulgated a regulation under clause (A)(i), shall be authorized and may be made with respect to a food if—

"(i) a scientific body of the United States Government with official responsibility for public health protection or research directly relating to human nutrition (such as the National Institutes of Health or the Centers for Disease Control and Prevention) or the National Academy of Sciences or any of its subdivisions has published an authoritative statement, which is currently in effect, which identifies the nutrient level to which the claim refers;

"(ii) a person has submitted to the Secretary, at least 120 days (during which the Secretary may notify any person who is making a claim as authorized by clause (C) that such person has not submitted all the information required by such clause) before the first introduction into interstate commerce of the food with a label containing the claim, (I) a notice of the claim, which shall include the exact words used in the claim and shall include a concise description of the basis upon which such person relied for determining that the requirements of subclause (i) have been satisfied, (II) a copy of the statement referred to in subclause (i) upon which such person relied in making the claim, and (III) a balanced representation of the scientific literature relating to the nutrient level to which the claim refers;

"(iii) the claim and the food for which the claim is made are in compliance with clauses (A) and (B), and are otherwise in compliance with paragraph (a) and section 201(n); and

"(iv) the claim is stated in a manner so that the claim is an accurate representation of the authoritative statement referred to in subclause (i) and so that the claim enables the public to comprehend the information provided in the claim and to understand the relative significance of such information in the context of a total daily diet.

For purposes of this clause, a statement shall be regarded as an authoritative statement of a scientific body described in subclause (i) only if the statement is published by the scientific body and shall not include a statement of an employee of the scientific body made in the individual capacity of the employee.

"(H) A claim submitted under the requirements of clause (G) may be made until—

"(i) such time as the Secretary issues a regulation—

"(I) prohibiting or modifying the claim and the regulation has become effective, or

"(II) finding that the requirements of clause (G) have not been met, including finding that the petitioner had not submitted all the information required by such clause; or

"(ii) a district court of the United States in an enforcement proceeding under chapter III has determined that the requirements of clause (G) have not been met.".

SEC. 305. REFERRAL STATEMENTS.

Section 403(r)(2)(B) (21 U.S.C. 343(r)(2)(B)) is amended to read as follows:

"(B) If a claim described in subparagraph (1)(A) is made with respect to a nutrient in a food and the Secretary makes a determination that the food contains a nutrient at a level that increases to persons in the general population the risk of a disease or health-related condition that is diet related, the label or labeling of such food shall contain, prominently and in immediate proximity to such claim, the following statement: 'See nutrition information for ____ content.' The blank shall identify the nutrient associated with the increased disease or health-related condition risk. In making the determination described in this clause, the Secretary shall take into account the significance of the food in the total daily diet.".

SEC. 306. DISCLOSURE OF IRRADIATION.

Chapter IV (21 U.S.C. 341 et seq.) is amended by inserting after section 403B the following:

"DISCLOSURE

"SEC. 403C. (a) No provision of section 201(n), 403(a), or 409 21 USC 343–3. shall be construed to require on the label or labeling of a food a separate radiation disclosure statement that is more prominent than the declaration of ingredients required by section 403(i)(2).

"(b) In this section, the term 'radiation disclosure statement' means a written statement that discloses that a food has been intentionally subject to radiation.".

SEC. 307. IRRADIATION PETITION.

Not later than 60 days following the date of the enactment of this Act, the Secretary of Health and Human Services shall make a final determination on any petition pending with the Food and Drug Administration that would permit the irradiation of red meat under section 409(b)(1) of the Federal Food, Drug, and Cosmetic Act. If the Secretary does not make such determination, the Secretary shall, not later than 60 days following the date of the enactment of this Act, provide the Committee on Commerce of the House of Representatives and the Committee on Labor and Human Resources of the Senate an explanation of the process followed by the Food and Drug Administration in reviewing the petition referred to in paragraph (1) and the reasons action on the petition was delayed.

SEC. 308. GLASS AND CERAMIC WARE.   21 USC 348 note.

(a) IN GENERAL.—The Secretary may not implement any requirement which would ban, as an unapproved food additive, lead and cadmium based enamel in the lip and rim area of glass and ceramic ware before the expiration of one year after the date such requirement is published.

(b) LEAD AND CADMIUM BASED ENAMEL.—Unless the Secretary determines, based on available data, that lead and cadmium based enamel on glass and ceramic ware—

    (1) which has less than 60 millimeters of decorating area below the external rim, and

    (2) which is not, by design, representation, or custom of usage intended for use by children,

is unsafe, the Secretary shall not take any action before January 1, 2003, to ban lead and cadmium based enamel on such glass and ceramic ware. Any action taken after January 1, 2003, to ban such enamel on such glass and ceramic ware as an unapproved food additive shall be taken by regulation and such regulation shall provide that such products shall not be removed from the market before 1 year after publication of the final regulation.

SEC. 309. FOOD CONTACT SUBSTANCES.

(a) FOOD CONTACT SUBSTANCES.—Section 409(a) (21 U.S.C. 348(a)) is amended—
   (1) in paragraph (1)—
      (A) by striking "subsection (i)" and inserting "subsection (j)"; and
      (B) by striking at the end "or";
   (2) by striking the period at the end of paragraph (2) and inserting "; or";
   (3) by inserting after paragraph (2) the following:
"(3) in the case of a food additive as defined in this Act that is a food contact substance, there is—
      "(A) in effect, and such substance and the use of such substance are in conformity with, a regulation issued under this section prescribing the conditions under which such additive may be safely used; or
      "(B) a notification submitted under subsection (h) that is effective."; and
   (4) by striking the matter following paragraph (3) (as added by paragraph (3)) and inserting the following flush sentence: "While such a regulation relating to a food additive, or such a notification under subsection (h)(1) relating to a food additive that is a food contact substance, is in effect, and has not been revoked pursuant to subsection (i), a food shall not, by reason of bearing or containing such a food additive in accordance with the regulation or notification, be considered adulterated under section 402(a)(1).".

(b) NOTIFICATION FOR FOOD CONTACT SUBSTANCES.—Section 409 (21 U.S.C. 348), as amended by subsection (a), is further amended—
   (1) by redesignating subsections (h) and (i), as subsections (i) and (j), respectively;
   (2) by inserting after subsection (g) the following:

"Notification Relating to a Food Contact Substance

"(h)(1) Subject to such regulations as may be promulgated under paragraph (3), a manufacturer or supplier of a food contact substance may, at least 120 days prior to the introduction or delivery for introduction into interstate commerce of the food contact substance, notify the Secretary of the identity and intended use of the food contact substance, and of the determination of the manufacturer or supplier that the intended use of such food contact substance is safe under the standard described in subsection (c)(3)(A). The notification shall contain the information that forms the basis of the determination and all information required to be submitted by regulations promulgated by the Secretary.

"(2)(A) A notification submitted under paragraph (1) shall become effective 120 days after the date of receipt by the Secretary and the food contact substance may be introduced or delivered for introduction into interstate commerce, unless the Secretary makes a determination within the 120-day period that, based on the data and information before the Secretary, such use of the food contact substance has not been shown to be safe under the standard described in subsection (c)(3)(A), and informs the manufacturer or supplier of such determination.

"(B) A decision by the Secretary to object to a notification shall constitute final agency action subject to judicial review.

"(C) In this paragraph, the term 'food contact substance' means the substance that is the subject of a notification submitted under paragraph (1), and does not include a similar or identical substance manufactured or prepared by a person other than the manufacturer identified in the notification.

"(3)(A) The process in this subsection shall be utilized for authorizing the marketing of a food contact substance except where the Secretary determines that submission and review of a petition under subsection (b) is necessary to provide adequate assurance of safety, or where the Secretary and any manufacturer or supplier agree that such manufacturer or supplier may submit a petition under subsection (b).

"(B) The Secretary is authorized to promulgate regulations to identify the circumstances in which a petition shall be filed under subsection (b), and shall consider criteria such as the probable consumption of such food contact substance and potential toxicity of the food contact substance in determining the circumstances in which a petition shall be filed under subsection (b).

"(4) The Secretary shall keep confidential any information provided in a notification under paragraph (1) for 120 days after receipt by the Secretary of the notification. After the expiration of such 120 days, the information shall be available to any interested party except for any matter in the notification that is a trade secret or confidential commercial information.

"(5)(A)(i) Except as provided in clause (ii), the notification program established under this subsection shall not operate in any fiscal year unless—

"(I) an appropriation equal to or exceeding the applicable amount under clause (iv) is made for such fiscal year for carrying out such program in such fiscal year; and

"(II) the Secretary certifies that the amount appropriated for such fiscal year for the Center for Food Safety and Applied Nutrition of the Food and Drug Administration (exclusive of the appropriation referred to in subclause (I)) equals or exceeds the amount appropriated for the Center for fiscal year 1997, excluding any amount appropriated for new programs.

"(ii) The Secretary shall, not later than April 1, 1999, begin accepting and reviewing notifications submitted under the notification program established under this subsection if—

"(I) an appropriation equal to or exceeding the applicable amount under clause (iii) is made for the last six months of fiscal year 1999 for carrying out such program during such period; and

"(II) the Secretary certifies that the amount appropriated for such period for the Center for Food Safety and Applied Nutrition of the Food and Drug Administration (exclusive of the appropriation referred to in subclause (I)) equals or exceeds an amount equivalent to one-half the amount appropriated for the Center for fiscal year 1997, excluding any amount appropriated for new programs.

"(iii) For the last six months of fiscal year 1999, the applicable amount under this clause is $1,500,000, or the amount specified in the budget request of the President for the six-month period involved for carrying out the notification program in fiscal year 1999, whichever is less.

"(iv) For fiscal year 2000 and subsequent fiscal years, the applicable amount under this clause is $3,000,000, or the amount specified in the budget request of the President for the fiscal year involved for carrying out the notification program under this subsection, whichever is less.

"(B) For purposes of carrying out the notification program under this subsection, there are authorized to be appropriated such sums as may be necessary for each of the fiscal years 1999 through fiscal year 2003, except that such authorization of appropriations is not effective for a fiscal year for any amount that is less than the applicable amount under clause (iii) or (iv) of subparagraph (A), whichever is applicable.

"(C) Not later than April 1 of fiscal year 1998 and February 1 of each subsequent fiscal year, the Secretary shall submit a report to the Committees on Appropriations of the House of Representatives and the Senate, the Committee on Commerce of the House of Representatives, and the Committee on Labor and Human Resources of the Senate that provides an estimate of the Secretary of the costs of carrying out the notification program established under this subsection for the next fiscal year.

"(6) In this section, the term 'food contact substance' means any substance intended for use as a component of materials used in manufacturing, packing, packaging, transporting, or holding food if such use is not intended to have any technical effect in such food.";

(3) in subsection (i), as so redesignated by paragraph (1), by adding at the end the following: "The Secretary shall by regulation prescribe the procedure by which the Secretary may deem a notification under subsection (h) to no longer be effective."; and

(4) in subsection (j), as so redesignated by paragraph (1), by striking "subsections (b) to (h)" and inserting "subsections (b) to (i)".

TITLE IV—GENERAL PROVISIONS

SEC. 401. DISSEMINATION OF INFORMATION ON NEW USES.

(a) IN GENERAL.—Chapter V (21 U.S.C. 351 et seq.) is amended by inserting after subchapter C the following:

"SUBCHAPTER D—DISSEMINATION OF TREATMENT INFORMATION

21 USC 360aaa.

"SEC. 551. REQUIREMENTS FOR DISSEMINATION OF TREATMENT INFORMATION ON DRUGS OR DEVICES.

"(a) IN GENERAL.—Notwithstanding sections 301(d), 502(f), and 505, and section 351 of the Public Health Service Act (42 U.S.C. 262), a manufacturer may disseminate to—
        "(1) a health care practitioner;
        "(2) a pharmacy benefit manager;
        "(3) a health insurance issuer;
        "(4) a group health plan; or

"(5) a Federal or State governmental agency;
written information concerning the safety, effectiveness, or benefit
of a use not described in the approved labeling of a drug or device
if the manufacturer meets the requirements of subsection (b).

"(b) SPECIFIC REQUIREMENTS.—A manufacturer may disseminate information under subsection (a) on a new use only if—

"(1)(A) in the case of a drug, there is in effect for the
drug an application filed under subsection (b) or (j) of section
505 or a biologics license issued under section 351 of the Public
Health Service Act; or

"(B) in the case of a device, the device is being commercially
distributed in accordance with a regulation under subsection
(d) or (e) of section 513, an order under subsection (f) of such
section, or the approval of an application under section 515;

"(2) the information meets the requirements of section 552;

"(3) the information to be disseminated is not derived from
clinical research conducted by another manufacturer or if it
was derived from research conducted by another manufacturer,
the manufacturer disseminating the information has the
permission of such other manufacturer to make the dissemination;

"(4) the manufacturer has, 60 days before such dissemination, submitted to the Secretary—

"(A) a copy of the information to be disseminated;
and

"(B) any clinical trial information the manufacturer
has relating to the safety or effectiveness of the new use,
any reports of clinical experience pertinent to the safety
of the new use, and a summary of such information;

"(5) the manufacturer has complied with the requirements
of section 554 (relating to a supplemental application for such
use);

"(6) the manufacturer includes along with the information
to be disseminated under this subsection—

"(A) a prominently displayed statement that discloses—

"(i) that the information concerns a use of a drug
or device that has not been approved or cleared by
the Food and Drug Administration;

"(ii) if applicable, that the information is being
disseminated at the expense of the manufacturer;

"(iii) if applicable, the name of any authors of
the information who are employees of, consultants to,
or have received compensation from, the manufacturer,
or who have a significant financial interest in the
manufacturer;

"(iv) the official labeling for the drug or device
and all updates with respect to the labeling;

"(v) if applicable, a statement that there are products or treatments that have been approved or cleared
for the use that is the subject of the information being
disseminated pursuant to subsection (a)(1); and

"(vi) the identification of any person that has provided funding for the conduct of a study relating to
the new use of a drug or device for which such information is being disseminated; and

"(B) a bibliography of other articles from a scientific
reference publication or scientific or medical journal that

have been previously published about the use of the drug or device covered by the information disseminated (unless the information already includes such bibliography).

"(c) ADDITIONAL INFORMATION.—If the Secretary determines, after providing notice of such determination and an opportunity for a meeting with respect to such determination, that the information submitted by a manufacturer under subsection (b)(3)(B), with respect to the use of a drug or device for which the manufacturer intends to disseminate information, fails to provide data, analyses, or other written matter that is objective and balanced, the Secretary may require the manufacturer to disseminate—

"(1) additional objective and scientifically sound information that pertains to the safety or effectiveness of the use and is necessary to provide objectivity and balance, including any information that the manufacturer has submitted to the Secretary or, where appropriate, a summary of such information or any other information that the Secretary has authority to make available to the public; and

"(2) an objective statement of the Secretary, based on data or other scientifically sound information available to the Secretary, that bears on the safety or effectiveness of the new use of the drug or device.

21 USC
360aaa–1.

"SEC. 552. INFORMATION AUTHORIZED TO BE DISSEMINATED.

"(a) AUTHORIZED INFORMATION.—A manufacturer may disseminate information under section 551 on a new use only if the information—

"(1) is in the form of an unabridged—

"(A) reprint or copy of an article, peer-reviewed by experts qualified by scientific training or experience to evaluate the safety or effectiveness of the drug or device involved, which was published in a scientific or medical journal (as defined in section 556(5)), which is about a clinical investigation with respect to the drug or device, and which would be considered to be scientifically sound by such experts; or

"(B) reference publication, described in subsection (b), that includes information about a clinical investigation with respect to the drug or device that would be considered to be scientifically sound by experts qualified by scientific training or experience to evaluate the safety or effectiveness of the drug or device that is the subject of such a clinical investigation; and

"(2) is not false or misleading and would not pose a significant risk to the public health.

"(b) REFERENCE PUBLICATION.—A reference publication referred to in subsection (a)(1)(B) is a publication that—

"(1) has not been written, edited, excerpted, or published specifically for, or at the request of, a manufacturer of a drug or device;

"(2) has not been edited or significantly influenced by such a manufacturer;

"(3) is not solely distributed through such a manufacturer but is generally available in bookstores or other distribution channels where medical textbooks are sold;

"(4) does not focus on any particular drug or device of a manufacturer that disseminates information under section

551 and does not have a primary focus on new uses of drugs or devices that are marketed or under investigation by a manufacturer supporting the dissemination of information; and

"(5) presents materials that are not false or misleading.

"SEC. 553. ESTABLISHMENT OF LIST OF ARTICLES AND PUBLICATIONS DISSEMINATED AND LIST OF PROVIDERS THAT RECEIVED ARTICLES AND REFERENCE PUBLICATIONS.

21 USC 360aaa–2.

"(a) IN GENERAL.—A manufacturer may disseminate information under section 551 on a new use only if the manufacturer prepares and submits to the Secretary biannually—

"(1) a list containing the titles of the articles and reference publications relating to the new use of drugs or devices that were disseminated by the manufacturer to a person described in section 551(a) for the 6-month period preceding the date on which the manufacturer submits the list to the Secretary; and

"(2) a list that identifies the categories of providers (as described in section 551(a)) that received the articles and reference publications for the 6-month period described in paragraph (1).

"(b) RECORDS.—A manufacturer that disseminates information under section 551 shall keep records that may be used by the manufacturer when, pursuant to section 555, such manufacturer is required to take corrective action and shall be made available to the Secretary, upon request, for purposes of ensuring or taking corrective action pursuant to such section. Such records, at the Secretary's discretion, may identify the recipient of information provided pursuant to section 551 or the categories of such recipients.

"SEC. 554. REQUIREMENT REGARDING SUBMISSION OF SUPPLEMENTAL APPLICATION FOR NEW USE; EXEMPTION FROM REQUIREMENT.

21 USC 360aaa–3.

"(a) IN GENERAL.—A manufacturer may disseminate information under section 551 on a new use only if—

"(1)(A) the manufacturer has submitted to the Secretary a supplemental application for such use; or

"(B) the manufacturer meets the condition described in subsection (b) or (c) (relating to a certification that the manufacturer will submit such an application); or

"(2) there is in effect for the manufacturer an exemption under subsection (d) from the requirement of paragraph (1).

"(b) CERTIFICATION ON SUPPLEMENTAL APPLICATION; CONDITION IN CASE OF COMPLETED STUDIES.—For purposes of subsection (a)(1)(B), a manufacturer may disseminate information on a new use if the manufacturer has submitted to the Secretary an application containing a certification that—

"(1) the studies needed for the submission of a supplemental application for the new use have been completed; and

"(2) the supplemental application will be submitted to the Secretary not later than 6 months after the date of the initial dissemination of information under section 551.

"(c) CERTIFICATION ON SUPPLEMENTAL APPLICATION; CONDITION IN CASE OF PLANNED STUDIES.—

"(1) IN GENERAL.—For purposes of subsection (a)(1)(B), a manufacturer may disseminate information on a new use if—

"(A) the manufacturer has submitted to the Secretary an application containing—

"(i) a proposed protocol and schedule for conducting the studies needed for the submission of a supplemental application for the new use; and

"(ii) a certification that the supplemental application will be submitted to the Secretary not later than 36 months after the date of the initial dissemination of information under section 551 (or, as applicable, not later than such date as the Secretary may specify pursuant to an extension under paragraph (3)); and

"(B) the Secretary has determined that the proposed protocol is adequate and that the schedule for completing such studies is reasonable.

"(2) PROGRESS REPORTS ON STUDIES.—A manufacturer that submits to the Secretary an application under paragraph (1) shall submit to the Secretary periodic reports describing the status of the studies involved.

"(3) EXTENSION OF TIME REGARDING PLANNED STUDIES.— The period of 36 months authorized in paragraph (1)(A)(ii) for the completion of studies may be extended by the Secretary if—

"(A) the Secretary determines that the studies needed to submit such an application cannot be completed and submitted within 36 months; or

"(B) the manufacturer involved submits to the Secretary a written request for the extension and the Secretary determines that the manufacturer has acted with due diligence to conduct the studies in a timely manner, except that an extension under this subparagraph may not be provided for more than 24 additional months.

"(d) EXEMPTION FROM REQUIREMENT OF SUPPLEMENTAL APPLICATION.—

"(1) IN GENERAL.—For purposes of subsection (a)(2), a manufacturer may disseminate information on a new use if—

"(A) the manufacturer has submitted to the Secretary an application for an exemption from meeting the requirement of subsection (a)(1); and

"(B)(i) the Secretary has approved the application in accordance with paragraph (2); or

"(ii) the application is deemed under paragraph (3)(A) to have been approved (unless such approval is terminated pursuant to paragraph (3)(B)).

"(2) CONDITIONS FOR APPROVAL.—The Secretary may approve an application under paragraph (1) for an exemption if the Secretary makes a determination described in subparagraph (A) or (B), as follows:

"(A) The Secretary makes a determination that, for reasons defined by the Secretary, it would be economically prohibitive with respect to such drug or device for the manufacturer to incur the costs necessary for the submission of a supplemental application. In making such determination, the Secretary shall consider (in addition to any other considerations the Secretary finds appropriate)—

"(i) the lack of the availability under law of any period during which the manufacturer would have exclusive marketing rights with respect to the new use involved; and "(ii) the size of the population expected to benefit from approval of the supplemental application.

"(B) The Secretary makes a determination that, for reasons defined by the Secretary, it would be unethical to conduct the studies necessary for the supplemental application. In making such determination, the Secretary shall consider (in addition to any other considerations the Secretary finds appropriate) whether the new use involved is the standard of medical care for a health condition.

"(3) TIME FOR CONSIDERATION OF APPLICATION; DEEMED APPROVAL.—

"(A) IN GENERAL.—The Secretary shall approve or deny an application under paragraph (1) for an exemption not later than 60 days after the receipt of the application. If the Secretary does not comply with the preceding sentence, the application is deemed to be approved.

"(B) TERMINATION OF DEEMED APPROVAL.—If pursuant to a deemed approval under subparagraph (A) a manufacturer disseminates written information under section 551 on a new use, the Secretary may at any time terminate such approval and under section 555(b)(3) order the manufacturer to cease disseminating the information.

"(e) REQUIREMENTS REGARDING APPLICATIONS.—Applications under this section shall be submitted in the form and manner prescribed by the Secretary.

"SEC. 555. CORRECTIVE ACTIONS; CESSATION OF DISSEMINATION.

"(a) POSTDISSEMINATION DATA REGARDING SAFETY AND EFFECTIVENESS.—

21 USC 360aaa–4.

"(1) CORRECTIVE ACTIONS.—With respect to data received by the Secretary after the dissemination of information under section 551 by a manufacturer has begun (whether received pursuant to paragraph (2) or otherwise), if the Secretary determines that the data indicate that the new use involved may not be effective or may present a significant risk to public health, the Secretary shall, after consultation with the manufacturer, take such action regarding the dissemination of the information as the Secretary determines to be appropriate for the protection of the public health, which may include ordering that the manufacturer cease the dissemination of the information.

"(2) RESPONSIBILITIES OF MANUFACTURERS TO SUBMIT DATA.—After a manufacturer disseminates information under section 551, the manufacturer shall submit to the Secretary a notification of any additional knowledge of the manufacturer on clinical research or other data that relate to the safety or effectiveness of the new use involved. If the manufacturer is in possession of the data, the notification shall include the data. The Secretary shall by regulation establish the scope of the responsibilities of manufacturers under this paragraph, including such limits on the responsibilities as the Secretary determines to be appropriate.

Regulations.

"(b) CESSATION OF DISSEMINATION.—

"(1) FAILURE OF MANUFACTURER TO COMPLY WITH REQUIREMENTS.—The Secretary may order a manufacturer to cease the dissemination of information pursuant to section 551 if the Secretary determines that the information being disseminated does not comply with the requirements established in this subchapter. Such an order may be issued only after the Secretary has provided notice to the manufacturer of the intent of the Secretary to issue the order and (unless paragraph (2)(B) applies) has provided an opportunity for a meeting with respect to such intent. If the failure of the manufacturer constitutes a minor violation of this subchapter, the Secretary shall delay issuing the order and provide to the manufacturer an opportunity to correct the violation.

"(2) SUPPLEMENTAL APPLICATIONS.—The Secretary may order a manufacturer to cease the dissemination of information pursuant to section 551 if—

"(A) in the case of a manufacturer that has submitted a supplemental application for a new use pursuant to section 554(a)(1), the Secretary determines that the supplemental application does not contain adequate information for approval of the new use for which the application was submitted;

"(B) in the case of a manufacturer that has submitted a certification under section 554(b), the manufacturer has not, within the 6-month period involved, submitted the supplemental application referred to in the certification; or

"(C) in the case of a manufacturer that has submitted a certification under section 554(c) but has not yet submitted the supplemental application referred to in the certification, the Secretary determines, after an informal hearing, that the manufacturer is not acting with due diligence to complete the studies involved.

"(3) TERMINATION OF DEEMED APPROVAL OF EXEMPTION REGARDING SUPPLEMENTAL APPLICATIONS.—If under section 554(d)(3) the Secretary terminates a deemed approval of an exemption, the Secretary may order the manufacturer involved to cease disseminating the information. A manufacturer shall comply with an order under the preceding sentence not later than 60 days after the receipt of the order.

"(c) CORRECTIVE ACTIONS BY MANUFACTURERS.—

"(1) IN GENERAL.—In any case in which under this section the Secretary orders a manufacturer to cease disseminating information, the Secretary may order the manufacturer to take action to correct the information that has been disseminated, except as provided in paragraph (2).

"(2) TERMINATION OF DEEMED APPROVAL OF EXEMPTION REGARDING SUPPLEMENTAL APPLICATIONS.—In the case of an order under subsection (b)(3) to cease disseminating information, the Secretary may not order the manufacturer involved to take action to correct the information that has been disseminated unless the Secretary determines that the new use described in the information would pose a significant risk to the public health.

21 USC
360aaa–5.

"SEC. 556. DEFINITIONS.

"For purposes of this subchapter:

"(1) The term 'health care practitioner' means a physician, or other individual who is a provider of health care, who is licensed under the law of a State to prescribe drugs or devices.

"(2) The terms 'health insurance issuer' and 'group health plan' have the meaning given such terms under section 2791 of the Public Health Service Act.

"(3) The term 'manufacturer' means a person who manufactures a drug or device, or who is licensed by such person to distribute or market the drug or device.

"(4) The term 'new use'—

"(A) with respect to a drug, means a use that is not included in the labeling of the approved drug; and

"(B) with respect to a device, means a use that is not included in the labeling for the approved or cleared device.

"(5) The term 'scientific or medical journal' means a scientific or medical publication—

"(A) that is published by an organization—

"(i) that has an editorial board;

"(ii) that utilizes experts, who have demonstrated expertise in the subject of an article under review by the organization and who are independent of the organization, to review and objectively select, reject, or provide comments about proposed articles; and

"(iii) that has a publicly stated policy, to which the organization adheres, of full disclosure of any conflict of interest or biases for all authors or contributors involved with the journal or organization;

"(B) whose articles are peer-reviewed and published in accordance with the regular peer-review procedures of the organization;

"(C) that is generally recognized to be of national scope and reputation;

"(D) that is indexed in the Index Medicus of the National Library of Medicine of the National Institutes of Health; and

"(E) that is not in the form of a special supplement that has been funded in whole or in part by one or more manufacturers.

"SEC. 557. RULES OF CONSTRUCTION.

21 USC
360aaa–6.

"(a) UNSOLICITED REQUEST.—Nothing in section 551 shall be construed as prohibiting a manufacturer from disseminating information in response to an unsolicited request from a health care practitioner.

"(b) DISSEMINATION OF INFORMATION ON DRUGS OR DEVICES NOT EVIDENCE OF INTENDED USE.—Notwithstanding subsection (a), (f), or (o) of section 502, or any other provision of law, the dissemination of information relating to a new use of a drug or device, in accordance with section 551, shall not be construed by the Secretary as evidence of a new intended use of the drug or device that is different from the intended use of the drug or device set forth in the official labeling of the drug or device. Such dissemination shall not be considered by the Secretary as labeling, adulteration, or misbranding of the drug or device.

"(c) PATENT PROTECTION.—Nothing in section 551 shall affect patent rights in any manner.

"(d) AUTHORIZATION FOR DISSEMINATION OF ARTICLES AND FEES FOR REPRINTS OF ARTICLES.—Nothing in section 551 shall be construed as prohibiting an entity that publishes a scientific journal (as defined in section 556(5)) from requiring authorization from the entity to disseminate an article published by such entity or charging fees for the purchase of reprints of published articles from such entity.".

(b) PROHIBITED ACT.—Section 301 (21 U.S.C. 331), as amended by section 210, is amended by adding at the end the following:

"(z) The dissemination of information in violation of section 551.".

21 USC 360aaa note.

(c) REGULATIONS.—Not later than 1 year after the date of enactment of this Act, the Secretary of Health and Human Services shall promulgate regulations to implement the amendments made by this section.

21 USC 360aaa note.

(d) EFFECTIVE DATE.—The amendments made by this section shall take effect 1 year after the date of enactment of this Act, or upon the Secretary's issuance of final regulations pursuant to subsection (c), whichever is sooner.

21 USC 360aaa note.

(e) SUNSET.—The amendments made by this section cease to be effective September 30, 2006, or 7 years after the date on which the Secretary promulgates the regulations described in subsection (c), whichever is later.

21 USC 360aaa note.

(f) STUDIES AND REPORTS.—

(1) GENERAL ACCOUNTING OFFICE.—

(A) IN GENERAL.—The Comptroller General of the United States shall conduct a study to determine the impact of subchapter D of chapter V of the Federal Food, Drug, and Cosmetic Act, as added by this section, on the resources of the Department of Health and Human Services.

(B) REPORT.—Not later than January 1, 2002, the Comptroller General of the United States shall prepare and submit to the Committee on Labor and Human Resources of the Senate and the Committee on Commerce of the House of Representatives a report of the results of the study.

(2) DEPARTMENT OF HEALTH AND HUMAN SERVICES.—

(A) IN GENERAL.—In order to assist Congress in determining whether the provisions of such subchapter should be extended beyond the termination date specified in subsection (e), the Secretary of Health and Human Services shall, in accordance with subparagraph (B), arrange for the conduct of a study of the scientific issues raised as a result of the enactment of such subchapter including issues relating to—

(i) the effectiveness of such subchapter with respect to the provision of useful scientific information to health care practitioners;

(ii) the quality of the information being disseminated pursuant to the provisions of such subchapter;

(iii) the quality and usefulness of the information provided, in accordance with such subchapter, by the Secretary or by the manufacturer at the request of the Secretary; and

(iv) the impact of such subchapter on research in the area of new uses, indications, or dosages, particularly the impact on pediatric indications and rare diseases.

(3) PROCEDURE FOR STUDY.—

(A) IN GENERAL.—The Secretary shall request the Institute of Medicine of the National Academy of Sciences to conduct the study required by paragraph (2), and to prepare and submit the report required by subparagraph (B), under an arrangement by which the actual expenses incurred by the Institute of Medicine in conducting the study and preparing the report will be paid by the Secretary. If the Institute of Medicine is unwilling to conduct the study under such an arrangement, the Comptroller General of the United States shall conduct such study.

(B) REPORT.—Not later than September 30, 2005, the Institute of Medicine or the Comptroller General of the United States, as appropriate, shall prepare and submit to the Committee on Labor and Human Resources of the Senate, the Committee on Commerce of the House of Representatives, and the Secretary a report of the results of the study required by paragraph (2). The Secretary, after the receipt of the report, shall make the report available to the public.

SEC. 402. EXPANDED ACCESS TO INVESTIGATIONAL THERAPIES AND DIAGNOSTICS.

Chapter V (21 U.S.C. 351 et seq.), as amended in section 401, is further amended by adding at the end the following:

"SUBCHAPTER E—GENERAL PROVISIONS RELATING TO DRUGS AND DEVICES

"SEC. 561. EXPANDED ACCESS TO UNAPPROVED THERAPIES AND DIAGNOSTICS.

21 USC 360bbb.

"(a) EMERGENCY SITUATIONS.—The Secretary may, under appropriate conditions determined by the Secretary, authorize the shipment of investigational drugs or investigational devices for the diagnosis, monitoring, or treatment of a serious disease or condition in emergency situations.

"(b) INDIVIDUAL PATIENT ACCESS TO INVESTIGATIONAL PRODUCTS INTENDED FOR SERIOUS DISEASES.—Any person, acting through a physician licensed in accordance with State law, may request from a manufacturer or distributor, and any manufacturer or distributor may, after complying with the provisions of this subsection, provide to such physician an investigational drug or investigational device for the diagnosis, monitoring, or treatment of a serious disease or condition if—

"(1) the licensed physician determines that the person has no comparable or satisfactory alternative therapy available to diagnose, monitor, or treat the disease or condition involved, and that the probable risk to the person from the investigational drug or investigational device is not greater than the probable risk from the disease or condition;

"(2) the Secretary determines that there is sufficient evidence of safety and effectiveness to support the use of the investigational drug or investigational device in the case described in paragraph (1);

"(3) the Secretary determines that provision of the investigational drug or investigational device will not interfere with the initiation, conduct, or completion of clinical investigations to support marketing approval; and

"(4) the sponsor, or clinical investigator, of the investigational drug or investigational device submits to the Secretary a clinical protocol consistent with the provisions of section 505(i) or 520(g), including any regulations promulgated under section 505(i) or 520(g), describing the use of the investigational drug or investigational device in a single patient or a small group of patients.

"(c) TREATMENT INVESTIGATIONAL NEW DRUG APPLICATIONS AND TREATMENT INVESTIGATIONAL DEVICE EXEMPTIONS.—Upon submission by a sponsor or a physician of a protocol intended to provide widespread access to an investigational drug or investigational device for eligible patients (referred to in this subsection as an 'expanded access protocol'), the Secretary shall permit such investigational drug or investigational device to be made available for expanded access under a treatment investigational new drug application or treatment investigational device exemption if the Secretary determines that—

"(1) under the treatment investigational new drug application or treatment investigational device exemption, the investigational drug or investigational device is intended for use in the diagnosis, monitoring, or treatment of a serious or immediately life-threatening disease or condition;

"(2) there is no comparable or satisfactory alternative therapy available to diagnose, monitor, or treat that stage of disease or condition in the population of patients to which the investigational drug or investigational device is intended to be administered;

"(3)(A) the investigational drug or investigational device is under investigation in a controlled clinical trial for the use described in paragraph (1) under an investigational drug application in effect under section 505(i) or investigational device exemption in effect under section 520(g); or

"(B) all clinical trials necessary for approval of that use of the investigational drug or investigational device have been completed;

"(4) the sponsor of the controlled clinical trials is actively pursuing marketing approval of the investigational drug or investigational device for the use described in paragraph (1) with due diligence;

"(5) in the case of an investigational drug or investigational device described in paragraph (3)(A), the provision of the investigational drug or investigational device will not interfere with the enrollment of patients in ongoing clinical investigations under section 505(i) or 520(g);

"(6) in the case of serious diseases, there is sufficient evidence of safety and effectiveness to support the use described in paragraph (1); and

"(7) in the case of immediately life-threatening diseases, the available scientific evidence, taken as a whole, provides a reasonable basis to conclude that the investigational drug or investigational device may be effective for its intended use and would not expose patients to an unreasonable and significant risk of illness or injury.

A protocol submitted under this subsection shall be subject to the provisions of section 505(i) or 520(g), including regulations promulgated under section 505(i) or 520(g). The Secretary may inform national, State, and local medical associations and societies,

89

voluntary health associations, and other appropriate persons about the availability of an investigational drug or investigational device under expanded access protocols submitted under this subsection. The information provided by the Secretary, in accordance with the preceding sentence, shall be the same type of information that is required by section 402(j)(3) of the Public Health Service Act.

"(d) TERMINATION.—The Secretary may, at any time, with respect to a sponsor, physician, manufacturer, or distributor described in this section, terminate expanded access provided under this section for an investigational drug or investigational device if the requirements under this section are no longer met.

"(e) DEFINITIONS.—In this section, the terms 'investigational drug', 'investigational device', 'treatment investigational new drug application', and 'treatment investigational device exemption' shall have the meanings given the terms in regulations prescribed by the Secretary.".

SEC. 403. APPROVAL OF SUPPLEMENTAL APPLICATIONS FOR APPROVED PRODUCTS.

21 USC 371 note.

(a) STANDARDS.—Not later than 180 days after the date of enactment of this Act, the Secretary of Health and Human Services shall publish in the Federal Register standards for the prompt review of supplemental applications submitted for approved articles under the Federal Food, Drug, and Cosmetic Act (21 U.S.C. 301 et seq.) or section 351 of the Public Health Service Act (42 U.S.C. 262).

(b) GUIDANCE TO INDUSTRY.—Not later than 180 days after the date of enactment of this Act, the Secretary shall issue final guidances to clarify the requirements for, and facilitate the submission of data to support, the approval of supplemental applications for the approved articles described in subsection (a). The guidances shall—

(1) clarify circumstances in which published matter may be the basis for approval of a supplemental application;

(2) specify data requirements that will avoid duplication of previously submitted data by recognizing the availability of data previously submitted in support of an original application; and

(3) define supplemental applications that are eligible for priority review.

(c) RESPONSIBILITIES OF CENTERS.—The Secretary shall designate an individual in each center within the Food and Drug Administration (except the Center for Food Safety and Applied Nutrition) to be responsible for—

(1) encouraging the prompt review of supplemental applications for approved articles; and

(2) working with sponsors to facilitate the development and submission of data to support supplemental applications.

(d) COLLABORATION.—The Secretary shall implement programs and policies that will foster collaboration between the Food and Drug Administration, the National Institutes of Health, professional medical and scientific societies, and other persons, to identify published and unpublished studies that may support a supplemental application, and to encourage sponsors to make supplemental applications or conduct further research in support of a supplemental application based, in whole or in part, on such studies.

SEC. 404. DISPUTE RESOLUTION.

Subchapter E of chapter V, as added by section 402, is amended by adding at the end the following:

21 USC
360bbb–1.
Regulations.

"SEC. 562. DISPUTE RESOLUTION.

"If, regarding an obligation concerning drugs or devices under this Act or section 351 of the Public Health Service Act, there is a scientific controversy between the Secretary and a person who is a sponsor, applicant, or manufacturer and no specific provision of the Act involved, including a regulation promulgated under such Act, provides a right of review of the matter in controversy, the Secretary shall, by regulation, establish a procedure under which such sponsor, applicant, or manufacturer may request a review of such controversy, including a review by an appropriate scientific advisory panel described in section 505(n) or an advisory committee described in section 515(g)(2)(B). Any such review shall take place in a timely manner. The Secretary shall promulgate such regulations within 1 year after the date of the enactment of the Food and Drug Administration Modernization Act of 1997.".

SEC. 405. INFORMAL AGENCY STATEMENTS.

Section 701 (21 U.S.C. 371) is amended by adding at the end the following:

"(h)(1)(A) The Secretary shall develop guidance documents with public participation and ensure that information identifying the existence of such documents and the documents themselves are made available to the public both in written form and, as feasible, through electronic means. Such documents shall not create or confer any rights for or on any person, although they present the views of the Secretary on matters under the jurisdiction of the Food and Drug Administration.

"(B) Although guidance documents shall not be binding on the Secretary, the Secretary shall ensure that employees of the Food and Drug Administration do not deviate from such guidances without appropriate justification and supervisory concurrence. The Secretary shall provide training to employees in how to develop and use guidance documents and shall monitor the development and issuance of such documents.

"(C) For guidance documents that set forth initial interpretations of a statute or regulation, changes in interpretation or policy that are of more than a minor nature, complex scientific issues, or highly controversial issues, the Secretary shall ensure public participation prior to implementation of guidance documents, unless the Secretary determines that such prior public participation is not feasible or appropriate. In such cases, the Secretary shall provide for public comment upon implementation and take such comment into account.

"(D) For guidance documents that set forth existing practices or minor changes in policy, the Secretary shall provide for public comment upon implementation.

"(2) In developing guidance documents, the Secretary shall ensure uniform nomenclature for such documents and uniform internal procedures for approval of such documents. The Secretary shall ensure that guidance documents and revisions of such documents are properly dated and indicate the nonbinding nature of the documents. The Secretary shall periodically review all guidance documents and, where appropriate, revise such documents.

"(3) The Secretary, acting through the Commissioner, shall maintain electronically and update and publish periodically in the Federal Register a list of guidance documents. All such documents shall be made available to the public.

"(4) The Secretary shall ensure that an effective appeals mechanism is in place to address complaints that the Food and Drug Administration is not developing and using guidance documents in accordance with this subsection.

"(5) Not later than July 1, 2000, the Secretary after evaluating the effectiveness of the Good Guidance Practices document, published in the Federal Register at 62 Fed. Reg. 8961, shall promulgate a regulation consistent with this subsection specifying the policies and procedures of the Food and Drug Administration for the development, issuance, and use of guidance documents.". *Regulations.*

SEC. 406. FOOD AND DRUG ADMINISTRATION MISSION AND ANNUAL REPORT.

(a) MISSION.—Section 903 (21 U.S.C. 393) is amended—

(1) by redesignating subsections (b) and (c) as subsections (d) and (e), respectively; and

(2) by inserting after subsection (a) the following:

"(b) MISSION.—The Administration shall—

"(1) promote the public health by promptly and efficiently reviewing clinical research and taking appropriate action on the marketing of regulated products in a timely manner;

"(2) with respect to such products, protect the public health by ensuring that—

"(A) foods are safe, wholesome, sanitary, and properly labeled;

"(B) human and veterinary drugs are safe and effective;

"(C) there is reasonable assurance of the safety and effectiveness of devices intended for human use;

"(D) cosmetics are safe and properly labeled; and

"(E) public health and safety are protected from electronic product radiation;

"(3) participate through appropriate processes with representatives of other countries to reduce the burden of regulation, harmonize regulatory requirements, and achieve appropriate reciprocal arrangements; and

"(4) as determined to be appropriate by the Secretary, carry out paragraphs (1) through (3) in consultation with experts in science, medicine, and public health, and in cooperation with consumers, users, manufacturers, importers, packers, distributors, and retailers of regulated products.".

(b) ANNUAL REPORT.—Section 903 (21 U.S.C. 393), as amended by subsection (a), is further amended by adding at the end the following:

"(f) AGENCY PLAN FOR STATUTORY COMPLIANCE.—

"(1) IN GENERAL.—Not later than 1 year after the date of enactment of the Food and Drug Administration Modernization Act of 1997, the Secretary, after consultation with appropriate scientific and academic experts, health care professionals, representatives of patient and consumer advocacy groups, and the regulated industry, shall develop and publish in the Federal Register a plan bringing the Secretary into compliance with each of the obligations of the Secretary under this Act. The *Federal Register, publication.*

Secretary shall review the plan biannually and shall revise the plan as necessary, in consultation with such persons.

"(2) OBJECTIVES OF AGENCY PLAN.—The plan required by paragraph (1) shall establish objectives and mechanisms to achieve such objectives, including objectives related to—

"(A) maximizing the availability and clarity of information about the process for review of applications and submissions (including petitions, notifications, and any other similar forms of request) made under this Act;

"(B) maximizing the availability and clarity of information for consumers and patients concerning new products;

"(C) implementing inspection and postmarket monitoring provisions of this Act;

"(D) ensuring access to the scientific and technical expertise needed by the Secretary to meet obligations described in paragraph (1);

"(E) establishing mechanisms, by July 1, 1999, for meeting the time periods specified in this Act for the review of all applications and submissions described in subparagraph (A) and submitted after the date of enactment of the Food and Drug Administration Modernization Act of 1997; and

"(F) eliminating backlogs in the review of applications and submissions described in subparagraph (A), by January 1, 2000.

Federal Register, publication.

"(g) ANNUAL REPORT.—The Secretary shall annually prepare and publish in the Federal Register and solicit public comment on a report that—

"(1) provides detailed statistical information on the performance of the Secretary under the plan described in subsection (f);

"(2) compares such performance of the Secretary with the objectives of the plan and with the statutory obligations of the Secretary; and

"(3) identifies any regulatory policy that has a significant negative impact on compliance with any objective of the plan or any statutory obligation and sets forth any proposed revision to any such regulatory policy.".

SEC. 407. INFORMATION SYSTEM.

(a) AMENDMENT.—Chapter VII (21 U.S.C. 371 et seq.) is amended by adding at the end the following:

"SUBCHAPTER D—INFORMATION AND EDUCATION

21 USC 379k.

"SEC. 741. INFORMATION SYSTEM.

"The Secretary shall establish and maintain an information system to track the status and progress of each application or submission (including a petition, notification, or other similar form of request) submitted to the Food and Drug Administration requesting agency action.".

21 USC 379k note.

(b) REPORT.—Not later than 1 year after the date of enactment of this Act, the Secretary of Health and Human Services shall submit a report to the Committee on Labor and Human Resources of the Senate and the Committee on Commerce of the House of Representatives on the status of the system to be established under the amendment made by subsection (a), including the projected costs of the system and concerns about confidentiality.

SEC. 408. EDUCATION AND TRAINING.

(a) FOOD AND DRUG ADMINISTRATION.—Chapter VII (21 U.S.C. 371 et seq.), as amended by section 407, is further amended by adding at the end the following section:

"SEC. 742. EDUCATION.   21 USC 379*l*.

"(a) IN GENERAL.—The Secretary shall conduct training and education programs for the employees of the Food and Drug Administration relating to the regulatory responsibilities and policies established by this Act, including programs for—

"(1) scientific training;

"(2) training to improve the skill of officers and employees authorized to conduct inspections under section 704;

"(3) training to achieve product specialization in such inspections; and

"(4) training in administrative process and procedure and integrity issues.

"(b) INTRAMURAL FELLOWSHIPS AND OTHER TRAINING PROGRAMS.—The Secretary, acting through the Commissioner, may, through fellowships and other training programs, conduct and support intramural research training for predoctoral and postdoctoral scientists and physicians.".

(b) CENTERS FOR DISEASE CONTROL AND PREVENTION.—

(1) IN GENERAL.—Part B of title III of the Public Health Service Act is amended by inserting after section 317F (42 U.S.C. 247b–7) the following:

"SEC. 317G. FELLOWSHIP AND TRAINING PROGRAMS.   42 USC 247b–8.

"The Secretary, acting through the Director of the Centers for Disease Control and Prevention, shall establish fellowship and training programs to be conducted by such Centers to train individuals to develop skills in epidemiology, surveillance, laboratory analysis, and other disease detection and prevention methods. Such programs shall be designed to enable health professionals and health personnel trained under such programs to work, after receiving such training, in local, State, national, and international efforts toward the prevention and control of diseases, injuries, and disabilities. Such fellowships and training may be administered through the use of either appointment or nonappointment procedures.".

(2) EFFECTIVE DATE.—The amendment made by this sub-   42 USC 247b–8
section is deemed to have taken effect July 1, 1995.   note.

SEC. 409. CENTERS FOR EDUCATION AND RESEARCH ON THERAPEUTICS.

Title IX of the Public Health Service Act (42 U.S.C. 299 et seq.) is amended by adding at the end of part A the following new section:

"SEC. 905. DEMONSTRATION PROGRAM REGARDING CENTERS FOR   42 USC 299a–3.
EDUCATION AND RESEARCH ON THERAPEUTICS.

"(a) IN GENERAL.—The Secretary, acting through the Administrator and in consultation with the Commissioner of Food and Drugs, shall establish a demonstration program for the purpose of making one or more grants for the establishment and operation of one or more centers to carry out the activities specified in subsection (b).

"(b) REQUIRED ACTIVITIES.—The activities referred to in subsection (a) are the following:

"(1) The conduct of state-of-the-art clinical and laboratory research for the following purposes:

"(A) To increase awareness of—

"(i) new uses of drugs, biological products, and devices;

"(ii) ways to improve the effective use of drugs, biological products, and devices; and

"(iii) risks of new uses and risks of combinations of drugs and biological products.

"(B) To provide objective clinical information to the following individuals and entities:

"(i) Health care practitioners or other providers of health care goods or services.

"(ii) Pharmacy benefit managers.

"(iii) Health maintenance organizations or other managed health care organizations.

"(iv) Health care insurers or governmental agencies.

"(v) Consumers.

"(C) To improve the quality of health care while reducing the cost of health care through—

"(i) the appropriate use of drugs, biological products, or devices; and

"(ii) the prevention of adverse effects of drugs, biological products, and devices and the consequences of such effects, such as unnecessary hospitalizations.

"(2) The conduct of research on the comparative effectiveness and safety of drugs, biological products, and devices.

"(3) Such other activities as the Secretary determines to be appropriate, except that the grant may not be expended to assist the Secretary in the review of new drugs.

"(c) APPLICATION FOR GRANT.—A grant under subsection (a) may be made only if an application for the grant is submitted to the Secretary and the application is in such form, is made in such manner, and contains such agreements, assurances, and information as the Secretary determines to be necessary to carry out this section.

"(d) PEER REVIEW.—A grant under subsection (a) may be made only if the application for the grant has undergone appropriate technical and scientific peer review.

"(e) AUTHORIZATION OF APPROPRIATIONS.—For the purpose of carrying out this section, there are authorized to be appropriated $2,000,000 for fiscal year 1998, and $3,000,000 for each of fiscal years 1999 through 2002.".

SEC. 410. MUTUAL RECOGNITION AGREEMENTS AND GLOBAL HARMONIZATION.

(a) GOOD MANUFACTURING PRACTICE REQUIREMENTS.—Section 520(f)(1)(B) (21 U.S.C. 360j(f)(1)(B)) is amended—

(1) in clause (i), by striking ", and" at the end and inserting a semicolon;

(2) in clause (ii), by striking the period and inserting "; and"; and

(3) by inserting after clause (ii) the following:

"(iii) ensure that such regulation conforms, to the extent practicable, with internationally recognized standards defining quality systems, or parts of the standards, for medical devices.".

(b) HARMONIZATION EFFORTS.—Section 803 (21 U.S.C. 383) is amended by adding at the end the following:

"(c)(1) The Secretary shall support the Office of the United States Trade Representative, in consultation with the Secretary of Commerce, in meetings with representatives of other countries to discuss methods and approaches to reduce the burden of regulation and harmonize regulatory requirements if the Secretary determines that such harmonization continues consumer protections consistent with the purposes of this Act.

"(2) The Secretary shall support the Office of the United States Trade Representative, in consultation with the Secretary of Commerce, in efforts to move toward the acceptance of mutual recognition agreements relating to the regulation of drugs, biological products, devices, foods, food additives, and color additives, and the regulation of good manufacturing practices, between the European Union and the United States.

"(3) The Secretary shall regularly participate in meetings with representatives of other foreign governments to discuss and reach agreement on methods and approaches to harmonize regulatory requirements.

"(4) The Secretary shall, not later than 180 days after the date of enactment of the Food and Drug Administration Modernization Act of 1997, make public a plan that establishes a framework for achieving mutual recognition of good manufacturing practices inspections.

"(5) Paragraphs (1) through (4) shall not apply with respect to products defined in section 201(ff).".

SEC. 411. ENVIRONMENTAL IMPACT REVIEW.

Chapter VII (21 U.S.C. 371 et seq.), as amended by section 407, is further amended by adding at the end the following:

"SUBCHAPTER E—ENVIRONMENTAL IMPACT REVIEW

"SEC. 746. ENVIRONMENTAL IMPACT.

21 USC 379o.

"Notwithstanding any other provision of law, an environmental impact statement prepared in accordance with the regulations published in part 25 of title 21, Code of Federal Regulations (as in effect on August 31, 1997) in connection with an action carried out under (or a recommendation or report relating to) this Act, shall be considered to meet the requirements for a detailed statement under section 102(2)(C) of the National Environmental Policy Act of 1969 (42 U.S.C. 4332(2)(C)).".

SEC. 412. NATIONAL UNIFORMITY FOR NONPRESCRIPTION DRUGS AND COSMETICS.

(a) NONPRESCRIPTION DRUGS.—Chapter VII (21 U.S.C. 371 et seq.), as amended by section 411, is further amended by adding at the end the following:

"Subchapter F—National Uniformity for Nonprescription Drugs and Preemption for Labeling or Packaging of Cosmetics

21 USC 379r.   "SEC. 751. NATIONAL UNIFORMITY FOR NONPRESCRIPTION DRUGS.

"(a) In General.—Except as provided in subsection (b), (c)(1), (d), (e), or (f), no State or political subdivision of a State may establish or continue in effect any requirement—

"(1) that relates to the regulation of a drug that is not subject to the requirements of section 503(b)(1) or 503(f)(1)(A); and

"(2) that is different from or in addition to, or that is otherwise not identical with, a requirement under this Act, the Poison Prevention Packaging Act of 1970 (15 U.S.C. 1471 et seq.), or the Fair Packaging and Labeling Act (15 U.S.C. 1451 et seq.).

"(b) Exemption.—

"(1) In general.—Upon application of a State or political subdivision thereof, the Secretary may by regulation, after notice and opportunity for written and oral presentation of views, exempt from subsection (a), under such conditions as may be prescribed in such regulation, a State or political subdivision requirement that—

"(A) protects an important public interest that would otherwise be unprotected, including the health and safety of children;

"(B) would not cause any drug to be in violation of any applicable requirement or prohibition under Federal law; and

"(C) would not unduly burden interstate commerce.

"(2) Timely action.—The Secretary shall make a decision on the exemption of a State or political subdivision requirement under paragraph (1) not later than 120 days after receiving the application of the State or political subdivision under paragraph (1).

"(c) Scope.—

"(1) In general.—This section shall not apply to—

"(A) any State or political subdivision requirement that relates to the practice of pharmacy; or

"(B) any State or political subdivision requirement that a drug be dispensed only upon the prescription of a practitioner licensed by law to administer such drug.

"(2) Safety or effectiveness.—For purposes of subsection (a), a requirement that relates to the regulation of a drug shall be deemed to include any requirement relating to public information or any other form of public communication relating to a warning of any kind for a drug.

"(d) Exceptions.—

"(1) In general.—In the case of a drug described in subsection (a)(1) that is not the subject of an application approved under section 505 or section 507 (as in effect on the day before the date of enactment of the Food and Drug Administration Modernization Act of 1997) or a final regulation promulgated by the Secretary establishing conditions under which the drug is generally recognized as safe and effective and not misbranded, subsection (a) shall apply only with respect to a requirement of a State or political subdivision of a State that relates to the same subject as, but is different from or in addition to, or that is otherwise not identical with—

"(A) a regulation in effect with respect to the drug pursuant to a statute described in subsection (a)(2); or

"(B) any other requirement in effect with respect to the drug pursuant to an amendment to such a statute made on or after the date of enactment of the Food and Drug Administration Modernization Act of 1997.

"(2) STATE INITIATIVES.—This section shall not apply to a State requirement adopted by a State public initiative or referendum enacted prior to September 1, 1997.

"(e) NO EFFECT ON PRODUCT LIABILITY LAW.—Nothing in this section shall be construed to modify or otherwise affect any action or the liability of any person under the product liability law of any State.

"(f) STATE ENFORCEMENT AUTHORITY.—Nothing in this section shall prevent a State or political subdivision thereof from enforcing, under any relevant civil or other enforcement authority, a requirement that is identical to a requirement of this Act.".

(b) INSPECTIONS.—Section 704(a)(1) (21 U.S.C. 374(a)(1)) is amended by striking "prescription drugs" each place it appears and inserting "prescription drugs, nonprescription drugs intended for human use,".

(c) MISBRANDING.—Subparagraph (1) of section 502(e) (21 U.S.C. 352(e)(1)) is amended to read as follows:

"(1)(A) If it is a drug, unless its label bears, to the exclusion of any other nonproprietary name (except the applicable systematic chemical name or the chemical formula)—

"(i) the established name (as defined in subparagraph (3)) of the drug, if there is such a name;

"(ii) the established name and quantity or, if determined to be appropriate by the Secretary, the proportion of each active ingredient, including the quantity, kind, and proportion of any alcohol, and also including whether active or not the established name and quantity or if determined to be appropriate by the Secretary, the proportion of any bromides, ether, chloroform, acetanilide, acetophenetidin, amidopyrine, antipyrine, atropine, hyoscine, hyoscyamine, arsenic, digitalis, digitalis glucosides, mercury, ouabain, strophanthin, strychnine, thyroid, or any derivative or preparation of any such substances, contained therein, except that the requirement for stating the quantity of the active ingredients, other than the quantity of those specifically named in this subclause, shall not apply to nonprescription drugs not intended for human use; and

"(iii) the established name of each inactive ingredient listed in alphabetical order on the outside container of the retail package and, if determined to be appropriate by the Secretary, on the immediate container, as prescribed in regulation promulgated by the Secretary, except that nothing in this subclause shall be deemed to require that any trade secret be divulged, and except that the requirements of this subclause with respect to alphabetical order shall apply only to nonprescription drugs that are not also cosmetics and that this subclause shall not apply to nonprescription drugs not intended for human use.

"(B) For any prescription drug the established name of such drug or ingredient, as the case may be, on such label (and on any labeling on which a name for such drug or ingredient is used) shall be printed prominently and in type at least half as large as that used thereon for any proprietary name or designation for such drug or ingredient, except that to the extent that compliance with the requirements of subclause (ii) or (iii) of clause (A) or this clause is impracticable, exemptions shall be established by regulations promulgated by the Secretary.".

(d) COSMETICS.—Subchapter F of chapter VII, as amended by subsection (a), is further amended by adding at the end the following:

21 USC 379s.

"SEC. 752. PREEMPTION FOR LABELING OR PACKAGING OF COSMETICS.

"(a) IN GENERAL.—Except as provided in subsection (b), (d), or (e), no State or political subdivision of a State may establish or continue in effect any requirement for labeling or packaging of a cosmetic that is different from or in addition to, or that is otherwise not identical with, a requirement specifically applicable to a particular cosmetic or class of cosmetics under this Act, the Poison Prevention Packaging Act of 1970 (15 U.S.C. 1471 et seq.), or the Fair Packaging and Labeling Act (15 U.S.C. 1451 et seq.).

"(b) EXEMPTION.—Upon application of a State or political subdivision thereof, the Secretary may by regulation, after notice and opportunity for written and oral presentation of views, exempt from subsection (a), under such conditions as may be prescribed in such regulation, a State or political subdivision requirement for labeling or packaging that—

"(1) protects an important public interest that would otherwise be unprotected;

"(2) would not cause a cosmetic to be in violation of any applicable requirement or prohibition under Federal law; and

"(3) would not unduly burden interstate commerce.

"(c) SCOPE.—For purposes of subsection (a), a reference to a State requirement that relates to the packaging or labeling of a cosmetic means any specific requirement relating to the same aspect of such cosmetic as a requirement specifically applicable to that particular cosmetic or class of cosmetics under this Act for packaging or labeling, including any State requirement relating to public information or any other form of public communication.

"(d) NO EFFECT ON PRODUCT LIABILITY LAW.—Nothing in this section shall be construed to modify or otherwise affect any action or the liability of any person under the product liability law of any State.

"(e) STATE INITIATIVE.—This section shall not apply to a State requirement adopted by a State public initiative or referendum enacted prior to September 1, 1997.".

21 USC 393 note.

SEC. 413. FOOD AND DRUG ADMINISTRATION STUDY OF MERCURY COMPOUNDS IN DRUGS AND FOOD.

(a) LIST AND ANALYSIS.—The Secretary of Health and Human Services shall, acting through the Food and Drug Administration—

(1) compile a list of drugs and foods that contain intentionally introduced mercury compounds, and

(2) provide a quantitative and qualitative analysis of the mercury compounds in the list under paragraph (1).

The Secretary shall compile the list required by paragraph (1) within 2 years after the date of enactment of the Food and Drug Administration Modernization Act of 1997 and shall provide the analysis required by paragraph (2) within 2 years after such date of enactment.

(b) STUDY.—The Secretary of Health and Human Services, acting through the Food and Drug Administration, shall conduct a study of the effect on humans of the use of mercury compounds in nasal sprays. Such study shall include data from other studies that have been made of such use.

(c) STUDY OF MERCURY SALES.—

(1) STUDY.—The Secretary of Health and Human Services, acting through the Food and Drug Administration and subject to appropriations, shall conduct, or shall contract with the Institute of Medicine of the National Academy of Sciences to conduct, a study of the effect on humans of the use of elemental, organic, or inorganic mercury when offered for sale as a drug or dietary supplement. Such study shall, among other things, evaluate—

(A) the scope of mercury use as a drug or dietary supplement; and

(B) the adverse effects on health of children and other sensitive populations resulting from exposure to, or ingestion or inhalation of, mercury when so used.

In conducting such study, the Secretary shall consult with the Administrator of the Environmental Protection Agency, the Chair of the Consumer Product Safety Commission, and the Administrator of the Agency for Toxic Substances and Disease Registry, and, to the extent the Secretary believes necessary or appropriate, with any other Federal or private entity.

(2) REGULATIONS.—If, in the opinion of the Secretary, the use of elemental, organic, or inorganic mercury offered for sale as a drug or dietary supplement poses a threat to human health, the Secretary shall promulgate regulations restricting the sale of mercury intended for such use. At a minimum, such regulations shall be designed to protect the health of children and other sensitive populations from adverse effects resulting from exposure to, or ingestion or inhalation of, mercury. Such regulations, to the extent feasible, should not unnecessarily interfere with the availability of mercury for use in religious ceremonies.

SEC. 414. INTERAGENCY COLLABORATION.

Section 903 (21 U.S.C. 393), as amended by section 406, is further amended by inserting after subsection (b) the following:

"(c) INTERAGENCY COLLABORATION.—The Secretary shall implement programs and policies that will foster collaboration between the Administration, the National Institutes of Health, and other science-based Federal agencies, to enhance the scientific and technical expertise available to the Secretary in the conduct of the duties of the Secretary with respect to the development, clinical investigation, evaluation, and postmarket monitoring of emerging medical therapies, including complementary therapies, and advances in nutrition and food science.".

SEC. 415. CONTRACTS FOR EXPERT REVIEW.

Chapter IX (21 U.S.C. 391 et seq.), as amended by section 214, is further amended by adding at the end the following:

"SEC. 907. CONTRACTS FOR EXPERT REVIEW.   21 USC 397.

"(a) IN GENERAL.—

"(1) Authority.—The Secretary may enter into a contract with any organization or any individual (who is not an employee of the Department) with relevant expertise, to review and evaluate, for the purpose of making recommendations to the Secretary on, part or all of any application or submission (including a petition, notification, and any other similar form of request) made under this Act for the approval or classification of an article or made under section 351(a) of the Public Health Service Act (42 U.S.C. 262(a)) with respect to a biological product. Any such contract shall be subject to the requirements of section 708 relating to the confidentiality of information.

"(2) Increased efficiency and expertise through contracts.—The Secretary may use the authority granted in paragraph (1) whenever the Secretary determines that use of a contract described in paragraph (1) will improve the timeliness of the review of an application or submission described in paragraph (1), unless using such authority would reduce the quality, or unduly increase the cost, of such review. The Secretary may use such authority whenever the Secretary determines that use of such a contract will improve the quality of the review of an application or submission described in paragraph (1), unless using such authority would unduly increase the cost of such review. Such improvement in timeliness or quality may include providing the Secretary increased scientific or technical expertise that is necessary to review or evaluate new therapies and technologies.

"(b) Review of Expert Review.—

"(1) In general.—Subject to paragraph (2), the official of the Food and Drug Administration responsible for any matter for which expert review is used pursuant to subsection (a) shall review the recommendations of the organization or individual who conducted the expert review and shall make a final decision regarding the matter in a timely manner.

"(2) Limitation.—A final decision by the Secretary on any such application or submission shall be made within the applicable prescribed time period for review of the matter as set forth in this Act or in the Public Health Service Act (42 U.S.C. 201 et seq.).".

SEC. 416. PRODUCT CLASSIFICATION.

Subchapter E of chapter V, as amended by section 404, is further amended by adding at the end the following:

"SEC. 563. CLASSIFICATION OF PRODUCTS.

21 USC 360bbb–2.

"(a) Request.—A person who submits an application or submission (including a petition, notification, and any other similar form of request) under this Act for a product, may submit a request to the Secretary respecting the classification of the product as a drug, biological product, device, or a combination product subject to section 503(g) or respecting the component of the Food and Drug Administration that will regulate the product. In submitting the request, the person shall recommend a classification for the product, or a component to regulate the product, as appropriate.

"(b) Statement.—Not later than 60 days after the receipt of the request described in subsection (a), the Secretary shall determine the classification of the product under subsection (a), or the component of the Food and Drug Administration that will regulate the product, and shall provide to the person a written statement that identifies such classification or such component, and the reasons for such determination. The Secretary may not modify such statement except with the written consent of the person, or for public health reasons based on scientific evidence.

"(c) INACTION OF SECRETARY.—If the Secretary does not provide the statement within the 60-day period described in subsection (b), the recommendation made by the person under subsection (a) shall be considered to be a final determination by the Secretary of such classification of the product, or the component of the Food and Drug Administration that will regulate the product, as applicable, and may not be modified by the Secretary except with the written consent of the person, or for public health reasons based on scientific evidence.".

SEC. 417. REGISTRATION OF FOREIGN ESTABLISHMENTS.

Section 510(i) (21 U.S.C. 360(i)) is amended to read as follows:

"(i)(1) Any establishment within any foreign country engaged in the manufacture, preparation, propagation, compounding, or processing of a drug or a device that is imported or offered for import into the United States shall register with the Secretary the name and place of business of the establishment and the name of the United States agent for the establishment.

"(2) The establishment shall also provide the information required by subsection (j).

"(3) The Secretary is authorized to enter into cooperative arrangements with officials of foreign countries to ensure that adequate and effective means are available for purposes of determining, from time to time, whether drugs or devices manufactured, prepared, propagated, compounded, or processed by an establishment described in paragraph (1), if imported or offered for import into the United States, shall be refused admission on any of the grounds set forth in section 801(a).".

SEC. 418. CLARIFICATION OF SEIZURE AUTHORITY.

Section 304(d)(1) (21 U.S.C. 334(d)(1)) is amended—

(1) in the fifth sentence, by striking "paragraphs (1) and (2) of section 801(e)" and inserting "subparagraphs (A) and (B) of section 801(e)(1)"; and

(2) by inserting after the fifth sentence the following: "Any person seeking to export an imported article pursuant to any of the provisions of this subsection shall establish that the article was intended for export at the time the article entered commerce.".

SEC. 419. INTERSTATE COMMERCE.

Section 709 (21 U.S.C. 379a) is amended by striking "a device" and inserting "a device, food, drug, or cosmetic".

SEC. 420. SAFETY REPORT DISCLAIMERS.

Chapter VII (21 U.S.C. 371 et seq.), as amended by section 412, is further amended by adding at the end the following:

"SUBCHAPTER G—SAFETY REPORTS

"SEC. 756. SAFETY REPORT DISCLAIMERS.   21 USC 379v.

"With respect to any entity that submits or is required to submit a safety report or other information in connection with the safety of a product (including a product that is a food, drug, device, dietary supplement, or cosmetic) under this Act (and any release by the Secretary of that report or information), such report or information shall not be construed to reflect necessarily a conclusion by the entity or the Secretary that the report or information constitutes an admission that the product involved malfunctioned, caused or contributed to an adverse experience, or otherwise caused or contributed to a death, serious injury, or serious illness. Such an entity need not admit, and may deny, that the report or information submitted by the entity constitutes an admission that the product involved malfunctioned, caused or contributed to an adverse experience, or caused or contributed to a death, serious injury, or serious illness.".

SEC. 421. LABELING AND ADVERTISING REGARDING COMPLIANCE WITH STATUTORY REQUIREMENTS.

Section 301 (21 U.S.C. 331) is amended by striking paragraph (l).

21 USC 321 note.

SEC. 422. RULE OF CONSTRUCTION.

Nothing in this Act or the amendments made by this Act shall be construed to affect the question of whether the Secretary of Health and Human Services has any authority to regulate any tobacco product, tobacco ingredient, or tobacco additive. Such authority, if any, shall be exercised under the Federal Food, Drug, and Cosmetic Act as in effect on the day before the date of the enactment of this Act.

TITLE V—EFFECTIVE DATE

21 USC 321 note.

SEC. 501. EFFECTIVE DATE.

Except as otherwise provided in this Act, this Act and the amendments made by this Act, other than the provisions of and the amendments made by sections 111, 121, 125, and 307, shall take effect 90 days after the date of enactment of this Act.

Approved November 21, 1997.

LEGISLATIVE HISTORY—S. 830 (H.R. 1411):

HOUSE REPORTS: Nos. 105–310, accompanying H.R. 1411 (Comm. on Commerce) and 105–399 (Comm. of Conference).
SENATE REPORTS: No. 105–43 (Comm. on Labor and Human Resources).
CONGRESSIONAL RECORD, Vol. 143 (1997):
    Sept. 11, 16, 18, 19, 23, 24, considered and passed Senate.
    Oct. 7, considered and passed House, amended, in lieu of H.R. 1411.
    Nov. 9, Senate and House agreed to conference report.
WEEKLY COMPILATION OF PRESIDENTIAL DOCUMENTS, Vol. 33 (1997):
    Nov. 21, Presidential remarks.

○